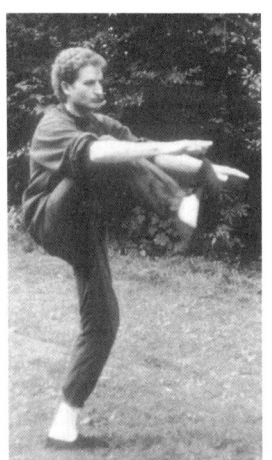

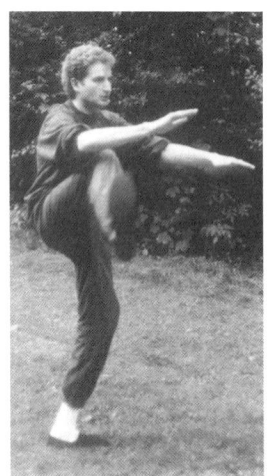

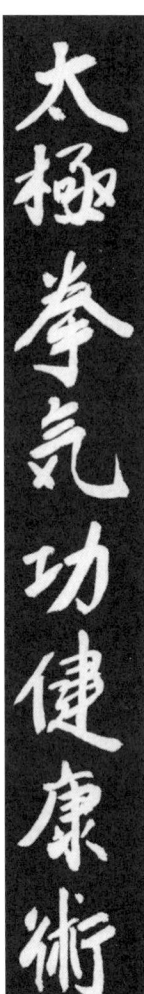

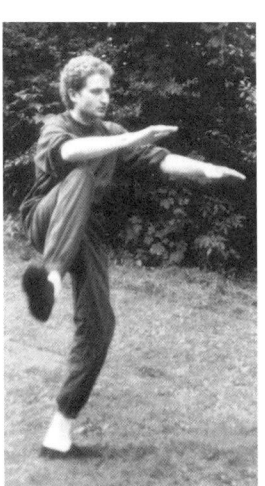

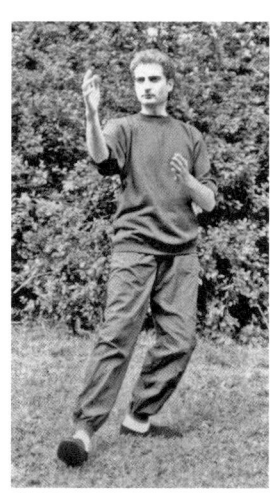

TAI CHI CHUAN
and
CHI KUNG

for
Health and Wellbeing

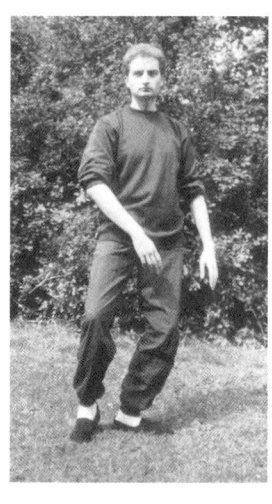

Glyn Williams

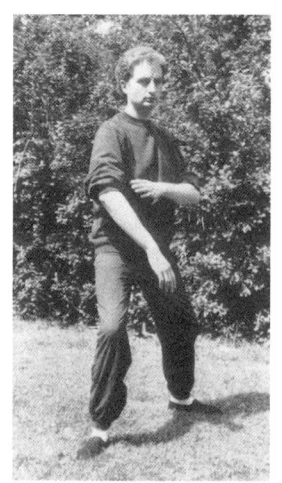

CHENG
MAN-CH'ING
Short Form

VG Productions

Cover design by Glyn Williams, Tristan Heath and Henryk Sienkiewicz
Illustration by Ilona Tate
Editorial advice Pat Walters, Val Reynolds and Lindsey Laing
Desktop publishing by Henryk Sienkiewicz
Calligraphy by Guey Ching Hwa
Cover photograph by Janet Adams
Technical advice and support by Tristan Heath of Heath IT Consulting
Published by VG Productions, UK

First Edition 2005

Printed by Antony Rowe Ltd UK

© 2005 Glyn Williams

All rights reserved. No part of this publication may be reproduced without written permission.

Glyn Williams asserts the moral right to be identified as the author of this book.

Any application of the techniques, ideas and suggestions in this book is at the reader's sole discretion and risk. It is advised that the reader should seek medical advice before beginning any physical exercise regime. The author and the publisher are not responsible whatsoever for any injury incurred by reading or following the instructions herein.

A catalogue record for this book is available from the British Library.

ISBN 1-874480-21-4

ACKNOWLEDGEMENTS

My thanks go to all those who have encouraged my enthusiasm and interest in T'ai Chi Ch'uan, Chi Kung and meditation, especially John Eastman, Ursula Smilde and Franklyn Sills.

I also would like to thank all those who have helped in the publication of this book, especially friends and students. These include Pat Walters, Val Reynolds, Sue Ellis, Janet Adams, Ilona Tate, Henry Goldstein, Henryk Sienkiewicz, Tristan Heath, Lindsey Robertson and many others too numerous to mention.

Glyn Williams.

FOREWORD

Writing this book comes from a desire to share with others some of the information I have been so fortunate to learn. This book has been written as a form of appreciation for all the tuition I have had over the years in T'ai chi and Chi Kung.

I feel very fortunate to have had such good tuition in T'ai chi and Chi Kung by sincere dedicated teachers, who themselves were able to find good teachers from various lineages. My desire and hope is that the knowledge in this book will fuel other people's interest in the subjects.

Glyn Williams
London, UK.
March 2005

CONTENTS

Acknowledgements
Forward
About the Author
Introduction

SECTION ONE   1

Chi Kung   3
Why Exercise?   4
Mind and Body   6
Traditional Chinese Medicine   7
T'ai Chi Ch'uan   9
Health and Wellbeing   11
Looking at Health   13
The Passage of Time   14
Stress Factors   15
About Stress   16
Meditation   17
What to do
About Meditation
Thoughts   18
Ways of Meditating
Ways of Focusing your Attention   19
When to Meditate
Where to Meditate
Who can Meditate
Self Sufficiency   20
Education   21
Self Knowledge   22

SECTION TWO   25

The Chinese Perspective   26
Chi Kung in China
Why Chi Kung?   27
Focus on the Form   28
Contemplate and Cultivate
Relaxation   29
How Chi Kung Works   30
Meditation Exercise   31
Relaxation Exercise   33

SECTION TWO Continued

Chi Kung Practice	34
Chi Kung Exercises	35
T'ai Chi Standing Postures	38
Ponder This	43

SECTION THREE   **47**

T'ai Chi Ch'uan - The benefits	49
Learning	51
Guidelines for Successful T'ai Chi Ch'uan Practice	52
Cheng Man-Ch'ing	57
Short Form Posture Names	60
Points to bear in Mind	63
Instructions for Learning the Form	64

SECTION FOUR   **127**

More on Exercise	129
Quality of Life	130
Advancing Years	
Reasons for Exercising	131
Benefits of T'ai Chi and Chi Kung	132
No Exercise	133
Adult Education	
The Teacher's Perspective	
The Learner's Role	134
The T'ai Chi Learning Environment	
The Teacher's Role	136
Personality and Character	137
Teaching	139
Learning	140
Intellectual Ability	141
Teacher's Observations	142
Personality Types	143
Motivation	143
Push Hands	144
In the Class	148
T'ai Chi Training	150
In Conclusion	164
Suggestions for Further Reading	166
Bibliography	167
Website Details	168

About the Author

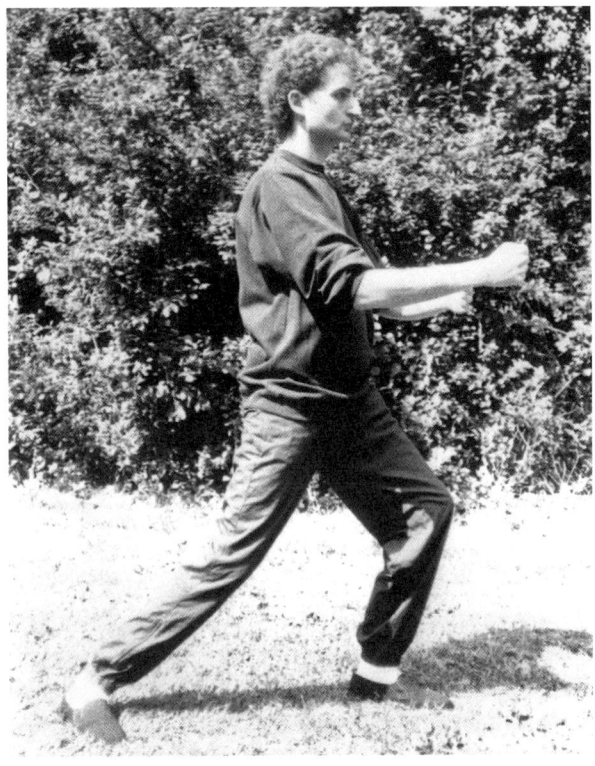

Glyn Williams has been practising T'ai Chi Ch'uan and Chi Kung since 1981. He initially studied the Yang long form with Ursula Smilde, she studied with Master Tang Liang Thia in Bangkok. He then went on to study the Cheng Man-Ch'ing short form with John Eastman, a direct student of Grandmaster Cheng when he taught in New York. Glyn also studied Chi Kung with Franklyn Sills who studied with several teachers including Fong Ha and Professor Yu Pen-Shi in San Francisco.

Glyn has been teaching T'ai chi and Chi Kung since 1988, having been qualified as an instructor by the T'ai Chi Union for Great Britain. Glyn runs residential retreats, teaches weekly group classes and offers individual tuition. He has been qualified as a teacher of the Alexander Technique since 1984 and teaches clients from all walks of life. He is also a freelance musician and teaches several musical instruments. Glyn has featured in radio and television programmes in connection with all aspects of his work.

Introduction

Forty years ago Chi Kung and T'ai chi were hardly known in the West. A few people practised these arts but they were not generally recognised. It could be said that the environment we create encourages the development of the resources needed to cope with that environment. On some level we need and want balance and harmony in our lives. People these days are familiar with Chi Kung and T'ai chi even if they do not practise them.

In China the practice of T'ai chi is encouraged as a way of coping with everyday life. T'ai chi and Chi Kung are seen as valuable assets to effective behaviour. In the West these arts are seen more as recreational and stress management techniques.

The western approach to exercise is more concerned with cardio-vascular fitness, muscular strength and general overall fitness and endurance. The oriental approach is concerned with building and conserving energy. They perceive everything as a manifestation of energy. The western approach of working harder and harder uses up energy; this can deplete the system and in some extreme cases can lead to burnout.

In China, people of all ages and physical conditions practise T'ai chi, Chi Kung and meditation to improve their frame of mind and body; as a result of building and circulating their energy. In the West, we have many de-energised, tense, angry people who would gain much benefit from learning these oriental approaches. The long-term benefits derived from practising these arts can significantly improve the quality of attention, co-ordination and physical responsiveness.

As a teacher, I think the most useful knowledge is anything that will enable people to create for themselves the life they want.

It is acknowledged that there is an increasing demand for home learning. Some people will naturally find it easier to study in their home environment. Some in rural settings live too far away from educational facilities; their only access to further learning is through correspondence courses and books.

I see this book as an important step in making these disciplines more accessible to the public. All the practices included in this book work directly or indirectly on our health and well-being. Education can never be undervalued. It is never too late to start learning. Why not begin to learn about these subjects now?

SECTION ONE

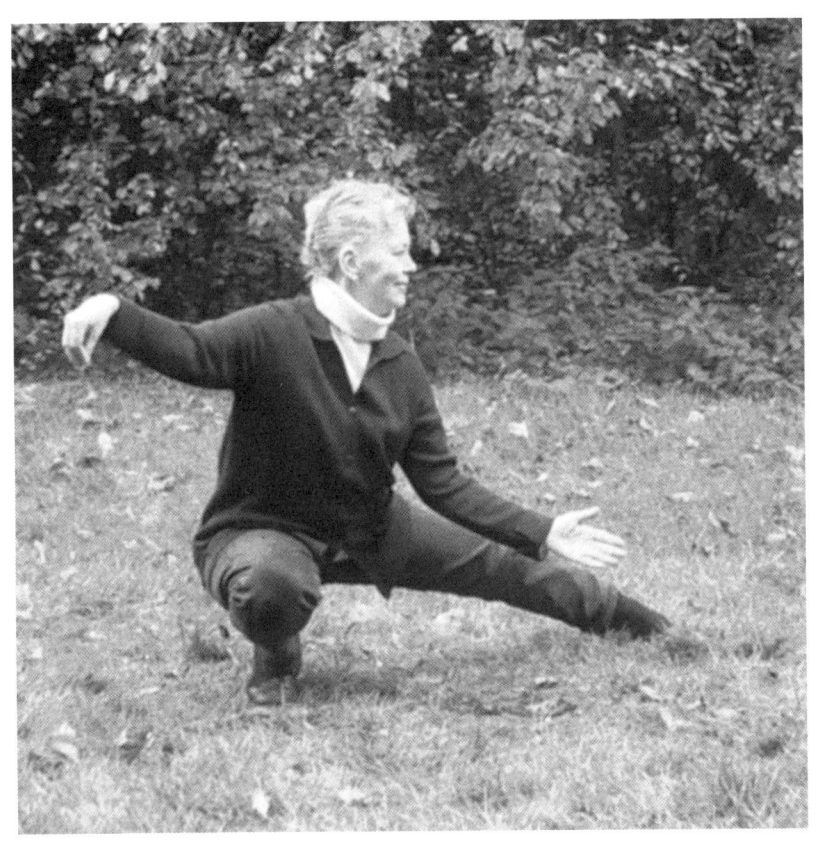

Chi Kung

The discipline of Chi Kung is one of the most ancient approaches to emerge from China. Chi Kung means work on energy. Chi is energy, Kung is work. The most famous teacher of Chi Kung was the Buddhist Monk named Bodhidarma, or as he was also called, Da Mo. He came from India to China during the Liang Dynasty (502-557 AD). He stayed for a period of time at the famous Shaolin Temple. He perceived the monks to be weak and sickly so he taught them exercises, which improved their health and increased their strength. Many styles of Martial Arts teach forms of Chi Kung in order to improve the effectiveness of their techniques. Currently there are innumerable styles and systems of Chi Kung taught all over the world. This is a far cry from past times when Chi Kung was a very secretive art. Only health related Chi Kung exercises were taught openly. In recent times books and publications have become more readily available on the subject, thus introducing Chi Kung to a wider audience.

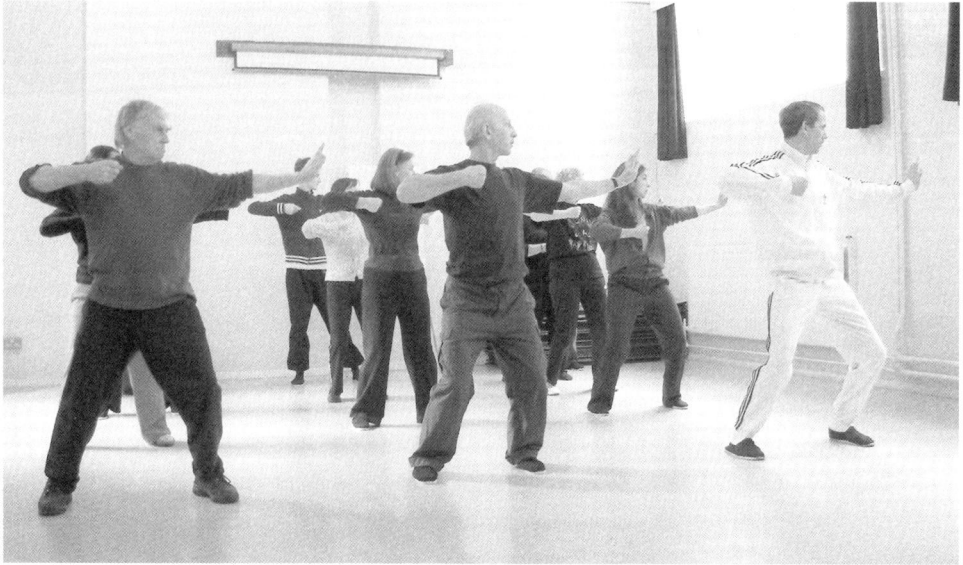

In Chinese health circles the opinion is that everything in life is a manifestation of energy. They believe illness to be caused by either a blockage in the body's energy system or insufficient energy in the system in the first place. By unblocking or increasing the energy good health is encouraged. The Chinese have studied energy for thousands of years. The cycles of nature were recorded in the 'I Ching' (Book of Changes, 1122BC). This was probably the first Chinese book written about Chi.

The writings of Lao Tzu who lived during the Jou dynasty (1122-934 BC) mention certain breathing techniques which would help people obtain good health. He wrote in his book 'Tao Te Ching':

Concentrate on Chi and achieve softness

This knowledge and understanding concerning energy has been understood for thousands of years in China. Surprisingly not many people know about it in the West. Only recently have books on the subject appeared in bookshops. Many, formerly secret documents have been published giving greater insight into this unique and ancient art.

We know that air, water, food and warmth are needed to sustain life. The Chinese believe that Chi is also needed; without it our body's battery runs down. The most effective way of keeping a car battery charged is to drive the car periodically. Similarly, physical stimulation is for the human body the easiest method of building energy (Chi).

Millions of people practise Chi Kung and T'ai chi in China every day. In England one occasionally sees people in the park doing some form of Chinese health exercise. More knowledge and tuition is needed over here. Hopefully, in the future our parks will also be full of people practising many diverse exercise forms.

Why Exercise?

The human body is designed for movement, therefore exercising on a regular basis is essential for our wellbeing. It is important that everyone be involved in some form of exercise routine. During exercise the heart is encouraged to work harder and beat faster, which results in a lower heart rate when the body is at rest. A conditioned heart holds a greater volume of blood and when it contracts it empties more thoroughly. In order to function properly, our bodies need a good, steady and consistent supply of blood. This provides our muscles with the necessary supplies of oxygen and nourishment.

How we breathe is very important. The way we breathe can have a profound effect on how we feel. Breathing properly increases our energy and relaxes one. Oxygen is sucked into the lungs on the in breath and gases containing carbon dioxide from the tissues are sent out on the out breath. The rhythmic inflation and deflation of the lungs is maintained by the movement of the ribcage and diaphragm. Better breathing means a better and healthier life. Efficient breathing is encouraged by physical exercise, where the demand on the muscles increases the intake of oxygen, causing the breath to become deeper and sometimes faster.

The medical establishment recognizes that the lack of physical exercise can lead to thinning and weakening of the bones. The legs are perceived as being very important in the Chinese approach. The emphasis is on keeping the legs active and strong. Exercises that encourage leg loading are approved of in western medical circles, as power and strength emanates from the legs.

The constant slow motion shifting of weight from leg to leg in Chi Kung and T'ai chi is an effective form of exercise, as it slowly increases muscle loading without stress. This gradually increases the strength of bones. The inside structure of a bone consists of tiny intersecting plates, mostly arranged in spiral patterns. These support the dense and thin pipe-like layer of bone called the cortical bone. Spiral forms inside the bone develop in response to the demand and stress placed on the bones by the loads they carry.

The gentle spiralling and rhythmic movements of the Chi Kung and T'ai chi forms help relax the muscles. This increases circulation to all muscle groups, joints and internal organs. The increased circulation improves the transport of oxygen and nutrients to the cells, tissues, muscles and bones.

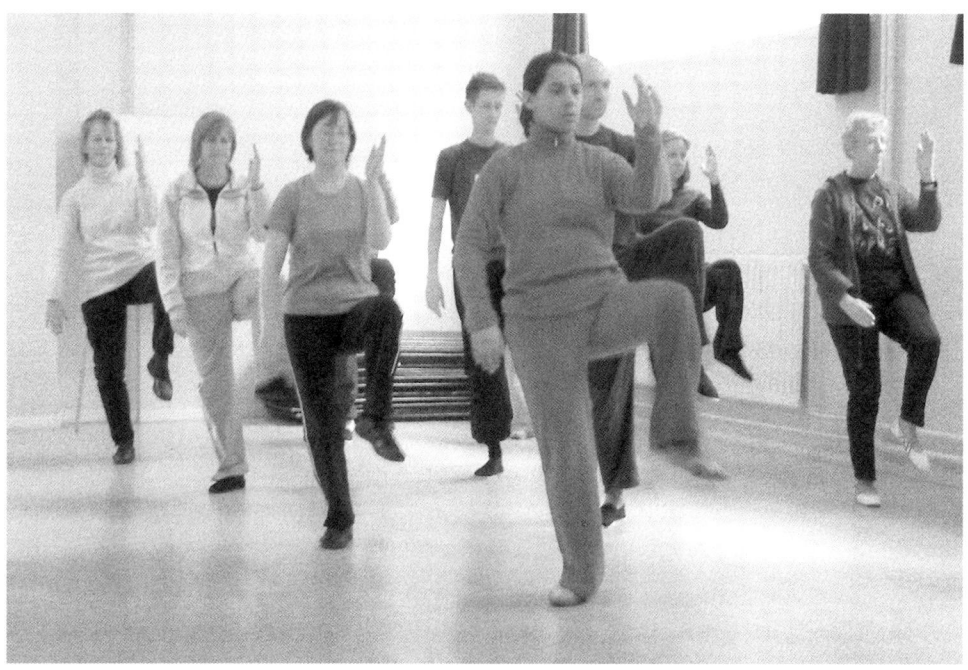

Chi Kung and T'ai chi movements are effective in lubricating cartilaginous joint surfaces through the process of rotation and compression. The compression is as a result of the slow movements being done with the knees bent; the turning of the hips creates the rotation. The great advantage of Chi Kung and T'ai chi is that their slow rhythmic movements enable people of all ages to improve their physical condition. Challenges placed on the legs create demands on the heart and lungs. Circulation improves and breathing becomes more relaxed and deeper. This whole condition helps reduce high blood pressure, decrease fatigue and develop endurance.

Mind and Body

The effect of exercise has also been observed in modern accelerated learning techniques. It has been discovered that children and adults have more propensity for mental activity if there is good blood circulation in the body. This leads to more oxygen being sent to the brain. Some exercises which involve left hand/right leg and right hand/left leg co-ordination may help children be more intelligent. Chi Kung and T'ai chi fit these criteria perfectly.

Sport in school is often only perceived from a competitive point of view and not as a supplement to mental capacity. There is too often a divide between mind and body in education, where each is seen as separate and taught as such. Students are not encouraged to see how each affects the other. I see my role in teaching as bridging the gap between mind and body. Tony Buzan, in his book, Use Your Head, mentions that we only use 4% of our brain's capacity. If we used 7% we would be geniuses. What could then be achieved if we used the other 93%?

In the Orient, people are able to do logic defying acts because they have delved deeper into the mind/body relationship. Our greater mind may be more than our capacity for logic. Through the practice of meditation people are able to quieten their thought processes and delve deeper into their greater mind, thus accessing more of their potential.

In the oriental approach the individual is seen as a microcosm of the universe. What happens within us affects the outer world and what happens in the universe affects the individual. By developing ourselves we can affect others and our environment. The more we know about ourselves the more potential we have for understanding others.

Traditional Chinese Medicine

Traditional Chinese Medicine (TCM) incorporates various approaches such as Acupuncture, Herbal Medicine, Chi Kung for self-healing as well as for healing others.

TCM is an important part of the health care system in China. In the West it may be difficult for some people to understand the theory and practice of TCM. It needs to be assessed in relation to the merits of its successful clinical results. Modern science requires everything to be proven by science. This may not always be possible. It should be realised that TCM predates western medicine by thousands of years, and it may be too sophisticated a system to be understood from a western viewpoint.

Acupuncture is more widely accepted in the West, especially by the medical profession. The American public was fascinated when James Renton of the New York Times when accompanying President Nixon on a trip to China in the early 1970s developed appendicitis, and was treated by acupuncture. Acupuncture however is only one aspect of the TCM system.

Julia J Tsuei writes in: 'Engineering in Medicine and Biology Magazine' Vol. 15, No 3, May/June 1996:

> ...Both of the above explanations are attempts to use structures and concepts acceptable to the mainstream medical community to explain acupuncture. But in grafting acupuncture to western medical theory, aspects foreign to orthodox medicine are simply jettisoned. Because of the emphasis on genetics, anatomy, physiology, and biochemistry in modern medicine, and a near complete denial of energetic processes in the body, chi (body energy) and meridians (paths of body energy flow) are either ignored or considered fallacies with some metaphorical or pneumonic value. Emphasis is placed by most researchers on the needle and the physical effect of its insertion into the skin, but this side of acupuncture is not essential. According to our research, acupuncture is essentially manipulation of bodily energy as it flows through the meridian system. The acupuncture needle is only one of many possible tools used to accomplish this activity...

> ...According to traditional Chinese medicine, a form of bodily energy, called chi, is generated in internal organs and systems. This energy combines with the breath and circulates throughout the body, forming paths called meridians. The meridians form a complex multi-level network that connects the various areas of the body, including the surface with the internal. All the various meridian systems work together to assure the flow and distribution of the chi throughout the body, thus controlling all bodily functions. The interwoven meridian system and the possibilities for diagnosis and treatment they offer are called meridian theory.

Later on in the same magazine Tsuei, in conjunction with F. M. K. Lam and Pesus Chou, goes on to write:

> ...Like acupuncture, the ancient practice of Chi Kung meditation is also based on meridian theory ...

> ...This practice supposedly improves the circulation of both blood and chi energy. Intermediate practitioners of Chi Kung begin to learn how to consciously monitor the flow of chi through their bodies. Very advanced practitioners and masters can control and emit chi that can be measured by some scientific devices. Emitted chi is said to have curative powers and can be used therapeutically ...

> ...Measurement readings, in particular chi points representing circulation, improved significantly after just half an hour of Chi Kung meditation. The whole body benefits from Chi Kung meditation, though there is an immediate clear effect on circulation. All bodily systems are interrelated and positive and negative affects on one system eventually effect other parts of the body.

T'ai Chi Ch'uan

T'ai Chi Ch'uan is generally acknowledged to have been created as a Martial Art. These days its popularity as a form of exercise is mainly attributed to its beneficial effects on health, fitness and wellbeing. T'ai chi's exact origin is unclear and unsubstantiated. An accepted theory about its origin is that a martial artist and Toaist priest by the name of Chang San-Feng, born in the 13th century, was seeking to create a new Martial Art. As he watched a snake and crane fighting he came to a realisation about circles and circular motion and how they could be applied in fighting situations. He observed the snake coiling in a circular manner away from the direct line of the crane's repeated attacks. It is said that from this enlightening moment came the formulation and creation of what is now called T'ai Chi Ch'uan.

T'ai chi these days is one of the most practised forms of exercise in the world. Parks in China and other eastern countries can be seen full of people practising various T'ai chi styles and forms. In the West, T'ai chi is gaining in popularity. Classes, clubs and adult education courses are seen more frequently. Forty years ago people may not have known what T'ai chi was; these days most people, including children, have heard of it and have a basic understanding of what it is.

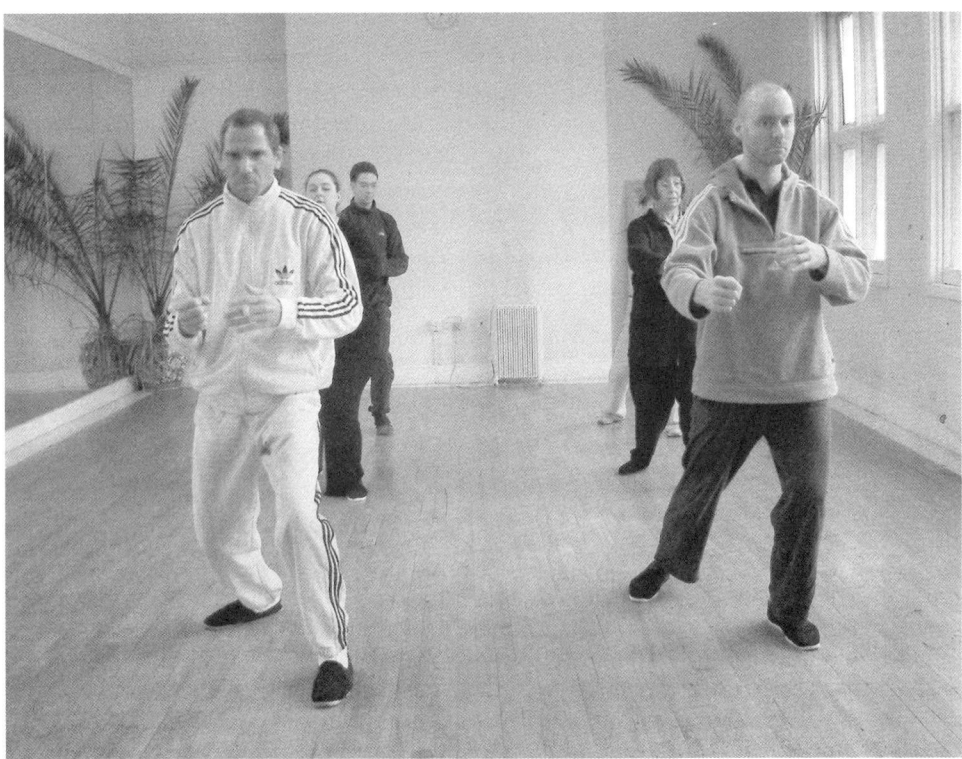

Many styles of T'ai chi have emerged and been created over the years. T'ai chi's exact history, from its perhaps mythological origin to now, is rather obscure. There is tangible evidence of the presence of T'ai chi for at least 400 years. We know that T'ai chi was taught in the Chen village, Wen county, Henan province in central China in the 1600's. Chen Wang Ting (1597-1664) taught T'ai chi in the Chen village. It's not known if he created the form or learned it elsewhere. The T'ai chi form was taught as a secret within the Chen family through oral transmission over the years. Only family members and some disciples from outside the family were taught, in a secretive, cloistered environment. This particular Chen style is generally acknowledged to be the first style of T'ai chi developed but it is not known if it resembles what Chang San-Feng, if he existed, created.

The other styles of T'ai chi practised all over the world are said to owe their origin to the Chen style whether directly of indirectly. Some people studied with the Chen family and then created their own styles. Over time new forms came out of these styles as people experimented with concepts and ideas. There seem to be as many interpretations of the various T'ai chi styles as there are practitioners. People bring their own experiences, aptitudes, desires and needs into the equation.

There is a certain uniformity of opinion about the principles and general ideas involved within the art of T'ai Chi Ch'uan. Most observers will recognize if someone is practising T'ai chi or not, as there is a similarity to all the diverse forms. Many of the styles though, do have their own unique character and a particular way of performing the movements.

Certain family forms may be better at achieving specific goals, for example martial effectiveness, health giving benefits and meditational skills. All the different styles have the above-mentioned potentials. The individual's focus, aim and desire affects the outcome.

Much is written about the founders of the new styles that have germinated out of the Chen form. The Yang style founder was Yang Lu Chuan (1799-1872). There are different versions of how he learned the Chen style. It was not initially from formal training but by spying on the Chen community doing their practice. Once caught he was brought in front of the Chen family master Chen Chang Hsing (1771-1853) to be punished. Yang was asked to show what he had learned. The level he had attained was higher than some of the Chen family members. He was then accepted as a student where he was taught formally in the Chen tradition.

Having completed his studies he then went on and taught and developed his own style, the Yang tradition. He became an accomplished martial artist and acquired the nickname of 'Yang the Invincible'. He taught his sons T'ai chi and they also became formidable fighters.

The Yang form of T'ai chi has become one of the most widely practised forms worldwide, mainly as a result of Yang Lu Chuan's grandson, Yang Cheng Fu (1883-1936). He altered some aspects of the family system. He slowed down the performance speed of the movements; he also made the transition between the movements more even. He removed the fast elements of the form as well as making the movements larger. All these factors made the form more accessible to the general public. The slow evenness of the movements had beneficial health effects, which also helped the form's popularity. The teaching of T'ai chi was at that time more open than it had been previously. This allowed more students access to the art which again helped in the expansion of T'ai chi.

One of the many students who studied with Yang Cheng Fu was Cheng Man-Ch'ing (1901-1975); he helped introduce T'ai chi to the West. Cheng's style is now a recognised style in its own right with great practitioners and teachers world wide popularising this unique form of exercise even further.

Health and Wellbeing

Cheng Man-Ch'ing claimed that our health is the most vital asset we possess; without it we are limited enormously. He felt that health education should be an important aspect of any curriculum planning programme. He stated that without good health, what use are we to our kith and kin, our family or our country? Often in schools the games period is the only physical activity programmed into the curriculum. The emphasis of the classes is on sport, competition and fitness. The presumption is that all of these will improve health and wellbeing.

People generally concern themselves with their health when they are having difficulties. Health care programmes are currently fairly abundant in adult education facilities. Their popularity is ever increasing in large cities and built up areas where there is greater potential for stress. People are becoming more aware that their working and living environment has an effect on their state of mind and body.

Our environment affects our personality. Personality is the way we see ourselves, or the way we are seen by others. Our personality has an effect on how we respond to the world. Practising T'ai chi, Chi Kung as well as meditation affects the practitioner's mind and body. Our nature changes, our perceptions change. The disciplines we practise affect our inner state.

Our thoughts affect our behaviour. The structure of our thought process affects our actions. Our thoughts precede our actions. Yet our behaviour is not set in stone. We all have the capacity to learn and change. This is why education is such a wonderful thing. We are able to go beyond our current limitations by learning.

The educational benefit of these arts happens when the mind is quietened. When the mind is quiet, our capacity to absorb information is greater because we are not interfering with the process of perception.

Sotto (1997) says:

> ... *We do not have to do anything in order to understand. All we have to do is to come to that which is to be understood with an open mind; to immerse ourselves by degree in it; to be patient; and to allow the situation to unfold itself.*

It is now agreed that inactivity or a sedentary life style could contribute to heart disease. Clinical studies in China have shown that the practice of T'ai chi and Chi Kung has a beneficial effect on blood pressure improving circulation throughout the muscular system. Care of the heart, as we have seen, is a crucial element in body maintenance. As your heart gets stronger through regular exercise, it pumps more blood with less effort, enabling you to exercise for longer periods. T'ai chi and Chi Kung, by their nature, are ideal health exercises as they are moderate and slow; they are always replenishing the body's reserves. The benefits of regular practice include an increase in the body's ability to resist illness and its resilience in relation to the external environment. Anyone can maintain a reasonable level of fitness through practising these arts. Age is no barrier to maintaining good physical condition. The movements of T'ai chi and Chi Kung, being soft, gentle and slow make them suitable for everyone, young and old.

Looking at Health

Health is generally defined as lack of disease or illness. In the Chinese approach, Chi (energy, bioelectricity) must flow in a balanced way throughout the body for good health to occur. Too much or too little Chi in any part of the body can lead to illness. Every cell in the body requires energy; if the supply becomes irregular then this can result in symptoms of sickness. In Chinese medicine it is said that you need to rebalance the Chi before you can cure the root of a disease, only then can you rebuild your physical strength and health. Chinese physicians believe that when the internal organs are healthy, the immune system will be stronger and the potential for resisting sickness will be higher.

Research has come up with some interesting observations. Dr. Yang (1989) writes:

> ...during the electrophysiological research of the 1960's several investigators discovered that bones are piezoelectric, that is when they are stressed, mechanical energy is converted to electrical energy in the form of electric current. This might explain one of the practices of Marrow Washing Chi Kung in which stress on the bones and muscles is increased in certain ways to increase the Chi circulation (electric circulation).

> ...It is presently believed that food and air are the fuel, which generates the electricity in the body through biochemical reaction. This electricity, which is circulated through the entire body through electrical conductive tissue, is one of the main energy sources, which keeps cells of the physical body alive. Whenever you have an injury or are sick, your body's electrical circulation is affected. If this circulation of electricity stops, you die. But bioelectric energy not only maintains life, it is also responsible for repairing physical damage.

> ...every cell of the body functions like an electric battery and is able to store electric charges.

...The flow of electricity can be reduced when muscles are tightened or the structure of the channels (the conductive tissue) is changed. In Chinese medicine this would be called Chi stagnation...

...Obviously, relaxation is able to increase electrical circulation.

The Passage of Time

Muscular strength, flexibility and stamina all tend to diminish with age, due not only to the natural shrinkage of muscles but also to the diminished capacity of the lungs to take in the oxygen needed to power the muscles. Although muscles tend to deteriorate with age at a faster rate than they are renewed, physical training nevertheless stimulates their build-up. As people are living longer, the elderly especially need to work on their health and wellbeing.

There is overwhelming proof that exercise decreases the risk of coronary artery disease, cancer and other diseases of life style. Regular moderate physical activity may perhaps extend the length and quality of life. The ancient Taoists were of this opinion. This is why they created certain Chi Kung exercises. In the last hundred years mankind and science have evolved at a tremendous rate. Still we have illness, disease, and wars. Perhaps we have not evolved on all levels. Being human, we have human foibles and failings. We are imperfect beings living in an imperfect realm. Our basest instincts some times come out, and we see the darker side of the human condition. On the other hand, we do have an amazing capacity to learn, to expand our potential and to develop all aspects of our being.

As psycho-physical organisms we need to be able to function effectively and consistently. The more knowledge we have about our own internal technology, the better off we will be in an ever-changing environment.

Stress Factors

The demands we encounter in society can often lead us in the direction of self-discovery, both mentally and physically. The demands placed upon us are ever increasing. People are always searching for ways to cope and redress the imbalances that are sometimes created.

Fear and worry are states that people experience often. Some people thrive on this, others find it detracts from their capacity. Some people spend most of their time in a state of fear of negative consequences. A friend's mother was asked why she worried so much. Her answer was, 'What would I do instead?' This is often the case for many people. They worry about how they look, their health, their finances, their family, their career, as well as other things.

Meyer Friedman and Ray Rosenman, who are two cardiologists, discovered that there is a link between emotional traits and heart disease. They categorised people into two types - type A and type B.

Type A behaviour patterns are characterised by:
- a sense of urgency
- free floating hostility
- doing two things at once
- impatience with others
- bossiness
- anger and hostility
- ambitiousness

Type B behaviour patterns are characterised by being:
- relaxed
- calm

Type A people gave more cause for concern as they had higher cholesterol levels, faster blood clotting times, higher adrenaline levels, more sudden deaths, and a sevenfold greater risk of heart disease. Reasons given for the causes of Type A were: peer pressure, parental expectations, high standards as well as cultural values of hard work and achievement.

It has been found that exercising helps de-stress Type A behaviour by reducing the physiological effects of stress. This is seen most in muscle relaxation. There are also psychological effects as a result of exercising. These are decreased levels of anxiety, stress and depression as well as increased emotional stability and wellbeing. There is also improvement in people's mood, self-esteem and self-concept. It is generally agreed that aerobic activity is successful at reducing cardiovascular reactivity to mental stress. I am of the opinion that exercises like Chi Kung and T'ai chi help reduce both the psychological and physiological effects of stress.

About Stress

Stress can be defined as an individual's response to stimuli perceived to be threatening, dangerous or overwhelming. Depending on your mental attitude and psychological state at any moment, anything can be a potential cause of stress: from an unexpectedly high telephone bill to having to cope with unwelcome relatives at Christmas. However a situation only consists of as many stressors as we choose to perceive. Two people faced with the same situation will probably perceive and respond to it differently. One person may see the situation as stressful, the other not. So how is it that the same situation is seen so differently? It is a function of the thought process of each individual, resulting in different points of view.

Stress is our way of reacting to situations based on what we see as reality. Some people say that there are times when a certain degree of stress can be useful to motivate us. Stress only becomes a problem when it reaches excessive levels where the demand exceeds our ability to respond or cope effectively. As a result of stress, certain negative reactions can be occurring in our bodies that may result in stress related symptoms and disorders.

Under stress the heart accelerates, breathing becomes shallower and faster, and muscles tense. Certain chemicals designed to mobilise one for 'fight or flight' are produced. These chemicals are designed to be dispersed but because of our sedentary lives we get less opportunity to burn them off. Physical exercise causes these stored products to be metabolised and cleared away.

Over the years the pace of life has increased. There is more pollution and over crowding in cities. Our minds are being influenced by the media. Our actions are being directed by the government and various institutions. We have societal expectations and obligations continually thrown in our face. We are bombarded by potential stressors all the time. How we respond to these affects our mind, body and emotions.

Current perception is that many of the illnesses in our modern society are as a result of our reaction to our circumstances. This culminates in certain situations becoming potential stressors. How we then cope with these gives us the impression of the degree of stress we experience. A valuable and useful counterbalance to stress is meditation.

Meditation

Meditation has been found to be an effective method for dealing with stress. For centuries people from different cultures all over the world have been practising various forms of meditative techniques. People have always been drawn to, or have searched for, some form of activity which will quieten their mind and give them peace. Meditational practices improve focus and concentration by quietening and freeing the mind of thoughts. The mind operates on many levels, yet most of us have been trained to use it only for thinking. In the past, people with insight discovered ways of operating in the world without having to use thought all the time. Obviously at times thoughts are useful. On other occasions they can be a burden, totally irrelevant, taking attention away from, and fragmenting our focus. Everyone can benefit from setting aside time every day to meditate, restoring balance to what may be a life filled with stress and tension.

What to Do

Now that we have discussed T'ai chi and Chi Kung history, theory and benefits, we need to look at how to practise these ancient arts, in order to get the most out of them. Mindless activity generally is of not much value. Therefore when doing any T'ai chi or Chi Kung movements you need to be mindful of what you are doing. Attention, focus and intention are all needed. One way of achieving this is through meditation.

About Meditation

A large component of T'ai chi and Chi Kung practice involves meditation. Through the practice of meditation you can learn to be more in the moment, more in the present. Thinking takes you away from experiencing the present moment. At any moment in your mind you can be in the past, present or future. Thinking about the argument you had with your boss first thing this morning is definitely a projection into the past. Thinking about where you could go with your partner for a meal this evening is definitely in the future. So when are you in the present? To be totally in the present you need complete awareness and focus without any thought.

Imagine you are a heart surgeon operating on a critical case. Allowing your mind to wander at the moment of incision would be totally inappropriate and possibly fatal. Your focus would need to be totally on what you are doing.

When sitting in meditation you will have the opportunity to observe your thoughts more clearly. Many of these thoughts go unnoticed by the conscious mind as they operate at a subconscious level.

Thoughts

Our thoughts can work for or against us. People often find themselves operating in a predictable, sometimes inappropriate manner resulting from thoughts adopted in the past. Their actions will be consistent with what they believe to be true, irrespective of how accurate their thoughts may be. Without looking or questioning their thought processes they may operate, to a certain degree, unaware of what they are doing.

Through practising meditation you become more attentive to your subconscious thoughts as they enter your awareness. You sometimes wonder where they come from as they dart in and out of your attention; some seem totally irrelevant appearing as if from nowhere, others may result from everyday worries and concerns. The more you meditate the more facility you develop for quietening and emptying your mind of irrelevant, distracting and sometimes disempowering thoughts.

Due to misconceptions and beliefs some people may have about their capacity to achieve what they want, they may not realise anything like their potential. Often they seldom realise the existence of such debilitating beliefs because they are submerged well below the level of consciousness. Meditation provides a constructive environment in which to observe and examine the validity of these beliefs. If you realise they are no longer true, you can then choose whether to hold on to them or let them go.

Ways of Meditating

There are various ways of meditating. You can be seated, standing, moving or lying down. When sitting you can be in the cross-legged 'lotus' position, in the Japanese 'sitting on the heels' position, or in a chair. It is important your back remains straight in whichever seated position you prefer. In standing meditation your back would be straight with your knees slightly bent, arms held away from your body.

Moving meditation would consist of a simple sequence of movements repeated for a period of time, with attention and focus. When meditating lying down, you would probably be in a supine position, that is, fully extended on your back, if possible with your head supported.

Ways of Focusing Your Attention

Each tradition has its preferred way of focusing attention. Some choose to focus on external objects such as a candle or a point on the ground. Some focus on the senses: what they see, hear, feel, smell, taste. Some focus on sounds that they create themselves, known as mantras. Others focus internally on themselves, on their breath and certain parts of their body. While others just focus on the thought process. Some people use music or natural sounds as a background for their meditation.

When to Meditate

With practice you could be in a meditative state of mind at any moment. To be able to get to that state, time will have to be set aside for regular practice. First thing in the morning is an ideal time for practice. Having just got out of bed your mind will be fairly quiet, so you have an immediate advantage. Last thing at night is also a good time, if you can prevent yourself from falling asleep. The length of your practice session could be increased gradually. When you practise regularly you naturally get into the appropriate frame of mind more quickly and easily each time.

Where to Meditate

In the initial stages where you practise is important. A quiet, pleasant environment free from disturbance is conducive to successful practice, although in time you will probably find you can meditate anywhere.

Who Can Meditate?

Anyone can meditate successfully. If you have an extremely busy lifestyle you may not be able to imagine sitting quietly devoid of thoughts. However, with correct practice you will begin to quieten and slow down your thinking process, until you are able to sit totally focused and attentive. Not only will you be training your focus to be on one thing at a time but more importantly you will be training your focus to be on what you want it to be on.

The more you practise, the more facility and ability you develop, which makes it easier for you to be totally focused without distraction. At that point it could be said you are in a state of meditation.

Meditation can be taken to different levels. Some people are happy enough to practise just to have a quiet mind so as not to be distracted in everyday activities. Others take it further in search of some truth or other, sitting patiently sometimes for hours every day for years waiting for enlightening moments.

If short periods of time could be found in the day to practise being quiet, you may observe a subsequent improvement in your approach to your activities: a calmer frame of mind and possibly a more relaxed body. Once your meditation routine is established you will find that your T'ai chi and Chi Kung practice will be more focused and relaxed. This will affect the flow of energy through your body as you do the movements.

Self Sufficiency

I think it is important to be self sufficient in relation to health and wellbeing. Often people create a dependency on others for their state of mind and body. In my own case I studied these arts so that I would not have to depend on anyone for my wellbeing. You can prepare a meal for someone or you can teach him or her how to cook. The latter, I feel, will be much more useful for the individual and will serve them throughout their life.

This moment now, is the beginning of our future. Our future is definitely influenced by our present. Now is the time to start taking care of ourselves. Prevention is far better than cure. Why create an environment for illness and disease? People often forget that they themselves are the environment for their own wellbeing.

Bruce Lee, the famous Martial Artist, said that if you have a question and you look at the question long enough, then the answer will appear. Perhaps the ancient oriental arts of T'ai chi and Chi Kung may be the answer to our current health related questions. These disciplines have been around for a very long time. In the past there were wise people in the East who knew how to maintain balance and wellbeing through the regulation of energy in the body. I think that these two arts are a legacy which can serve us equally well today in contemporary society.

Education

Education is an important aspect of everyone's life, as we are limited by what we do not know. We are also limited to what we know. This is why it is important to continue learning throughout our lives. 'In the land of the blind the one-eyed person is king'. This person has an enormous advantage over the others. It is also true to say that someone with greater knowledge and understanding has a distinct advantage. Information and knowledge can help people grow and advance. Life gets easier as they become more practical and efficient in their endeavours.

Teaching the oriental arts of Chi Kung and T'ai chi to western students has its challenges. Our approach and thinking differs quite a lot from the eastern approach. The Chinese are very advanced in their understanding of the relationship between mind and body. Their understanding of themselves and the universe is currently being proven by science. What they understand through meditation and observation we are confirming through scientific means. Zukav (1984) writes:

> ... The development of Buddhism shows that a profound and penetrating intellectual quest into the ultimate nature of reality can culminate in, or at least set the stage for, a quantum leap beyond rationality. In fact, on an individual level, this is one of the roads to enlightenment. Tibetan Buddhism calls it the Path without Form, or the Practice of Mind. The Path without Form is prescribed for people of intellectual temperament. The science of physics is following a similar path.
>
> The development of physics in the twentieth century already has transformed the consciousness of those involved with it. The study of complementarity, the uncertainty principle, quantum field theory and the Copenhagen Interpretation of Quantum Mechanics produces insights into the nature of reality very similar to those produced by the study of eastern philosophy.

In our society at the moment there is a need for the wisdom which was understood years ago in the Orient. I perceive my job of teaching these oriental arts as very important in this day and age, as these subjects are a means to re-establish balance and homeostasis for mind and body.

Self Knowledge

My Chi Kung instructor saw the teacher's role as a signpost, showing people the way without necessarily taking them there. The teacher teaches the subject in an enthusiastic way so as to encourage the student's interest in the subject. They then do the necessary work, in order to advance in their studies.

Teaching is important because the information you share with people may affect their subsequent lives. Our future has not been written yet and the seed for what ensues is in our present. We and our circumstances are the soil for the fruition of our future. Morea (1990) writes:

> *...each of us enters the world with potential for growth and, given the right soil, healthy growth will occur.*

Knowledge is only information. We need the wisdom to use knowledge wisely and appropriately for the good of ourselves and others. The decisions we make are affected by our desires and values. Our values are influenced by our morals. If we are not aware of our morals and values, then our decisions may be led by more basic animalistic tendencies. Holmes and Maclean (1992) write:

> *... Plato argued that wisdom was learned intuitively. The acquisition of knowledge was not logical, sequential and standardised as rationalists claimed but was the outcome of the interaction between the innate qualities of the learner and the potential sources of reinforcing morality in the texts. Since each individual might find different material appropriate to his or her moral development, the content of education should be selected in the light of individual differences.'*

Through the learning and practice of T'ai chi and Chi Kung we may develop higher morals and values which may be the deciding factors in us making wiser decisions about our actions for the future.

SECTION TWO

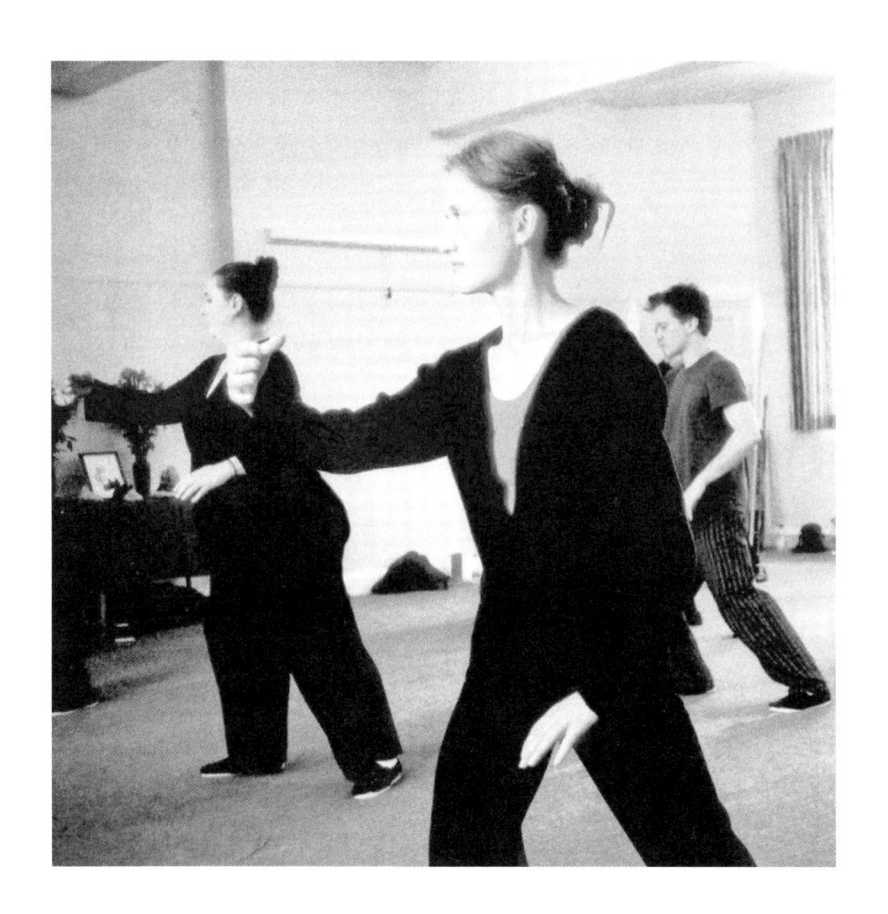

The Chinese Perspective

In the Chinese health system it is believed that one inherits a certain amount of energy from one's parents at birth; this is called prenatal Chi. This supply of energy is gradually used up throughout life. Some people inherit more than others do. The energy created by practising Chi Kung exercises adds to this existing level, helping to preserve natural vitality and youthfulness.

The ancient Taoists observed through their study that the aging process created certain conditions in people as well as nature. Among these were the loss of softness, pliability and vigour. The youthful qualities of liveliness, suppleness and flexibility were characteristics they sought to retain. They noticed children to be vibrant, malleable and energetic. They concluded that if the principles of youth could be maintained into advancing years, this would positively affect wellbeing.

A major factor in this equation from their perspective was energy. What was needed were ways of building up and storing energy. The Chi Kung exercises increased the level of energy and the ability to meditate helped conserve it. Many forms of Chi Kung are available to the general public. Some Chi Kung forms have been strongly discouraged in China as they are reported to affect mental stability. Their effect apparently is too strong for the human condition. In England, there are no reports of such conditions. Chi Kung forms are generally taught for either health/meditation or martial purposes. There is a growing trend for T'ai chi practitioners to be more interested in the martial aspects of their art. Their Chi Kung training reflects this tendency. Their emphasis is more on stamina, endurance and strength as a way of enhancing the effectiveness of their techniques. Historians are of the opinion that Chi Kung for health predates Chi Kung for martial purposes.

Chi Kung in China

Chi Kung practice involves a variety of exercises, some moving, some static, some sedentary. Many of these can be done focused on the breath or in co-ordination with breathing. Different exercises will work in different ways. Some exercises are designed to stimulate the energy, some to concentrate the energy, and some to circulate the energy. Understanding the purpose of the exercises helps deepen and expand the student's practice and experience.

China offers a comprehensive health care system. It is reported that there are approximately 2,100 traditional medicine hospitals and an estimated one million traditionally trained doctors and pharmacists throughout China. Chi Kung is one of the means for treating diseases in these hospitals.

People are now beginning to realise that combining aspects of western and Chinese medicine may be the least invasive and most beneficial therapy available for patients. Western doctors generally look for physical or chemical abnormalities in a patient, while Chinese doctors search for hidden forces that may be out of balance.

The Chinese government, in order to reduce the cost of health care, has encouraged people to take part in physical exercise routines as a way of lessening the burden on the state. This is also a way of encouraging people to look after and maintain their health. Reports state that there are millions of people who daily perform Chi Kung and T'ai chi exercises.

Why Chi Kung?

People come to Chi Kung for various reasons, to:

- manage stress
- increase energy level
- calm the mind
- relax the body
- satisfy curiosity and interest
- improve health
- deal with illness or recovery from physical discomfort

Chi Kung can be done for its own sake or for a reason. The reason could be: to be healthy, to be relaxed, to deal with illness or to remove discomfort. The reason may take you to a class or to buy a book, but when you practise Chi Kung, it is advisable that you do the exercises for their own sake. You need to place all your attention on what you are doing.

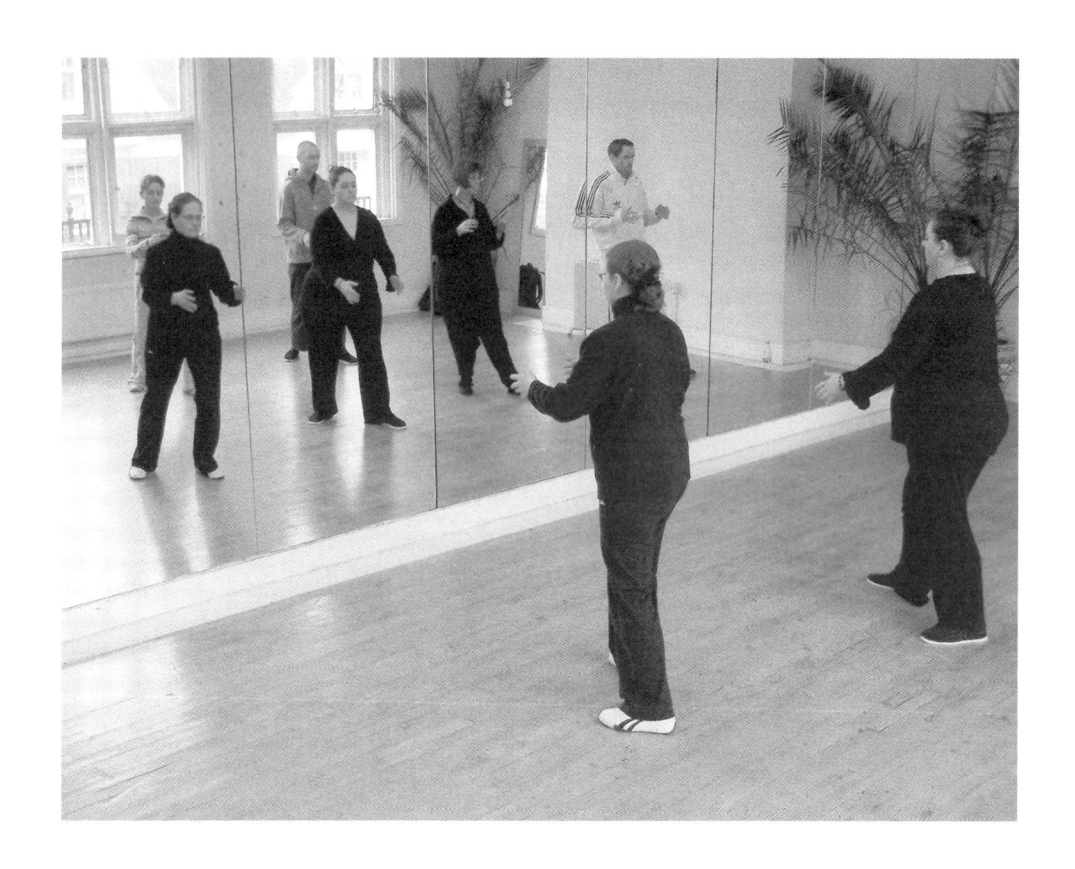

Focus on the Form

The form is the exercise you are doing. When you focus on the form you are focusing both on what you are doing as well as yourself. This on its own is meditation, which is the ability to bring total attention to what you are doing while you are doing it. If your mind wanders during any activity, then you may diminish the effectiveness of what you are doing. In relation to Chi Kung practice this can be seen as less return on your investment from an energy building point of view. The effect would be to diminish the potential level of energy attainable within your practice.

Contemplate and Cultivate

Chi Kung exercises help to stimulate, concentrate and circulate energy. Some exercises do more of one category than another. It is essential while doing Chi Kung practice to still the mind.

Chi follows Yi - Chi is energy, Yi is mind. Energy follows your intention and your attention. If the mind wanders energy is scattered. This is the importance in Chi

Kung of stilling and emptying the mind - it allows energy to be built and not wasted.

When practising Chi Kung movements the mind needs to be totally focused on the particular exercise that is being done. If at any point attention begins to wander, bring it back to the execution of the exercise. Over time one's attention will wander less. You will find that you can maintain extended periods of attention without thought. From a meditation point of view this is good practice. This will help your attention span and focus.

Relaxation

Relaxation refers to mind and body. Physical relaxation emanates from a certain mental state. The mind needs to be peaceful and calm as well as quiet. Tension, whether physical or mental, prevents us from doing our best. Learning to relax can help people be more aware of their body - this fact alone may help reduce the negative effects created by wear and tear.

- How relaxed do you feel at this moment, as you are reading this?
- On the scale of 0 -10. 10 being relaxed and 0 being tense, where do you find yourself generally?

In the Chinese approach to wellbeing, they say that tension interferes with the flow of energy in the body. It creates constriction in the musculature system that then interferes with blood circulation.

- Take a moment now to focus on your body.
- Using a gentle focus, wish for your muscles to become softer, freer and more relaxed.
- Continue these thoughts for a couple of minutes.
- Now wish/think for your whole body to become even softer, freer and more relaxed.

Directed focused thoughts have the capacity to influence one in the direction of one's thinking. The next time you feel tense or stressed, just take a couple of moments to focus on the whole body becoming softer, freer and more relaxed.

Practice leads to improvement. This applies to relaxation as much as to any other activity. Deeper relaxation can be achieved by setting aside time every day to lie down and consciously relax every part of your body. Spend anywhere in the region of ten to twenty minutes doing this. You will notice over time, that your normal state of being begins to become more relaxed, as your nervous system is being imbued with relaxed thoughts.

How Chi Kung Works

It could be said that with aging there may be a decline in vitality and energy levels. Chi Kung exercises are specifically designed to cultivate vitality and increase energy. This is without doubt a valuable resource as we work towards quality of life. The goal of cultivating energy is a means to improved health. The calmness created by doing the exercises will help focus the mind and encourage inner stillness.

It is believed that the relaxation and the slowness of the movements give Chi Kung its healing properties. Chi Kung forms are repetitive in nature. This fact alone helps lull the mind into stillness. The brainwave patterns slow down. This takes the brain into what is called alpha brainwave pattern. It has been discovered that in this state healing occurs within the body. Healers find that their brainwave activity naturally goes into this state when they heal.

When practising Chi Kung movements it is important to be mindful in each moment. When the Chi Kung movements are done with the mind focused on the process, the most positive effect is encouraged. Chi Kung encourages relaxation and an increase in energy; both these factors encourage improvement in the immune system's capacity to deal with the negative effects of stress. When practising, be relaxed and calm so as not to interfere with the flow of energy and blood circulation throughout the body.

The Chinese believe that there is a close relationship between the flow of blood and Chi. Warmth is generated as a result of the increased circulation and the flow of energy. It is said that where blood and warmth go, healing occurs. Performing any Chi Kung exercise facilitates the body's ability to heal itself.

Research in China has shown that physiological changes happen with Chi Kung practice. This is especially the case with the standing static exercises. There is a change in blood chemistry. There is a considerable increase in white blood cell count as well as in red blood cell count.

Meditation Exercise

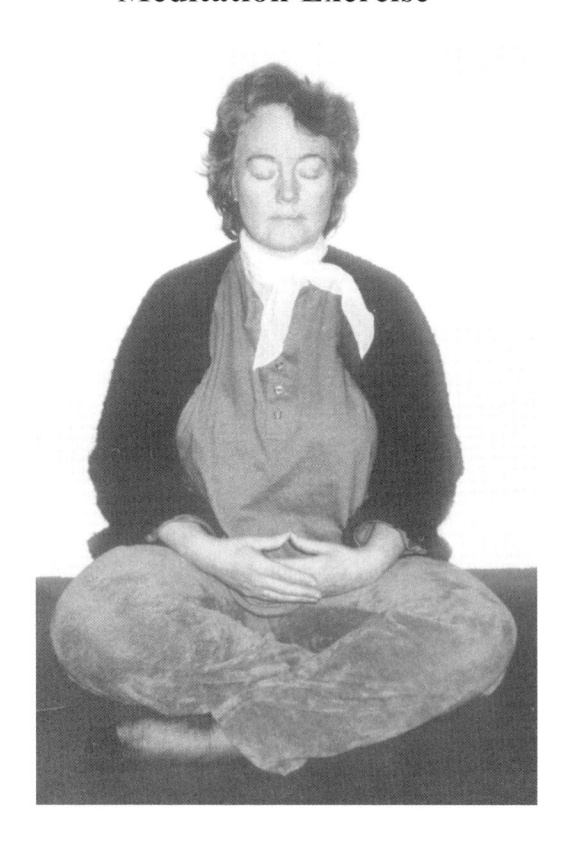

Sit upright, either on a chair, a kneeling stool, or cross-legged in a Lotus position on a cushion. It is preferable for the spine to be upright throughout any meditation session.

Sitting on a chair - If you are unfamiliar with meditating, you may prefer sitting on a chair. Keep you feet on the ground, about a foot apart. Do not lean back against the chair.

Sitting on a kneeling stool - You may prefer the Japanese zazen position, which is sitting on your heels. You can buy a wooden kneeling stool to sit on, to take the weight off your knees.

Sitting cross-legged in the Lotus position - Sitting on a firm cushion will help the cross-legged position as it raises your sitting bones above your heels, facilitating opening the hips without creating too much discomfort. You may want to rest against a wall. You may find the cross-legged position too uncomfortable to maintain. Work into it gradually; you may need to reposition yourself more than once during the session.

- Have the left hand resting on top of the right hand, with the tips of the thumbs touching. If sitting on a chair, you could have your hands resting on your knees or thighs.

- Have your tongue touching the roof of your mouth as if you are saying 'L'.

It is important in all the meditative postures to have your tongue touching the roof of your mouth - this connects the two main meridians in your body. This affects and changes the flow of energy in the body.

Steps to Meditation

1. Once you are sitting comfortably, bring your attention to the process of sitting.
2. Be aware of your thoughts, without being drawn into them. Notice as they come and go
3. Bring your attention to an area 2' to 3' below your navel, which is called the lower Tan Tien. Keep your attention gently focused there. If at any point your attention wanders, bring it back to focusing on your Tan Tien.

Any of these steps can be done for as short or as long a time period as you choose. Anywhere from five minutes to twenty minutes would be a good length of time to sit in meditation. Through the practice of a meditative technique, whether it be looking at a candle, chanting a mantra, focusing on your breath or a part of your body, you are beginning to train your mind to focus on one thing at a time which helps to minimise the distraction of thought. The more time spent practising, the more facility and ability is developed, which makes it even easier to meditate and sit for longer periods. This leads to more in depth understanding of what you are doing. When learning to meditate it is hard to keep your attention focused to start with. To train yourself to pay attention you can try narrowing your field of concentration to a category of objects first, where your mind still has some freedom of movement. If you find unwanted thoughts intruding, just keep bringing your attention back to the objects of concentration and you will find that your mind will become more focused. In the same way that focusing the rays of the sun with a magnifying glass makes them hot enough to burn paper, so focusing the scattered rays of thought makes the mind more penetrating and powerful. With the continued practice of meditation you may discover a greater sense of purpose and strength of will. Your thinking becomes clearer and more concentrated, affecting all that you do.

Relaxation Exercise

- Lie down either on the floor or on a bed so that you are totally flat. Have a pillow or some books under your head for support. Make sure that your arms and legs are uncrossed.
- Close your eyes. Allow your mind to be quiet and peaceful.
- Let all your weight rest on the ground.
- Allow your breathing to be comfortable and natural.
- Bring your attention to your body and begin to wish your muscles to be soft and relaxed.
- Allow your weight to sink deeper into the ground.
- Begin to let go of your body, as you give up responsibility to gravity.
- Allow your breathing to become relaxed.
- Allow your whole body to become relaxed and slightly heavier.
- Allow your weight to sink even more into the ground.
- Keep your mind quiet and relaxed.

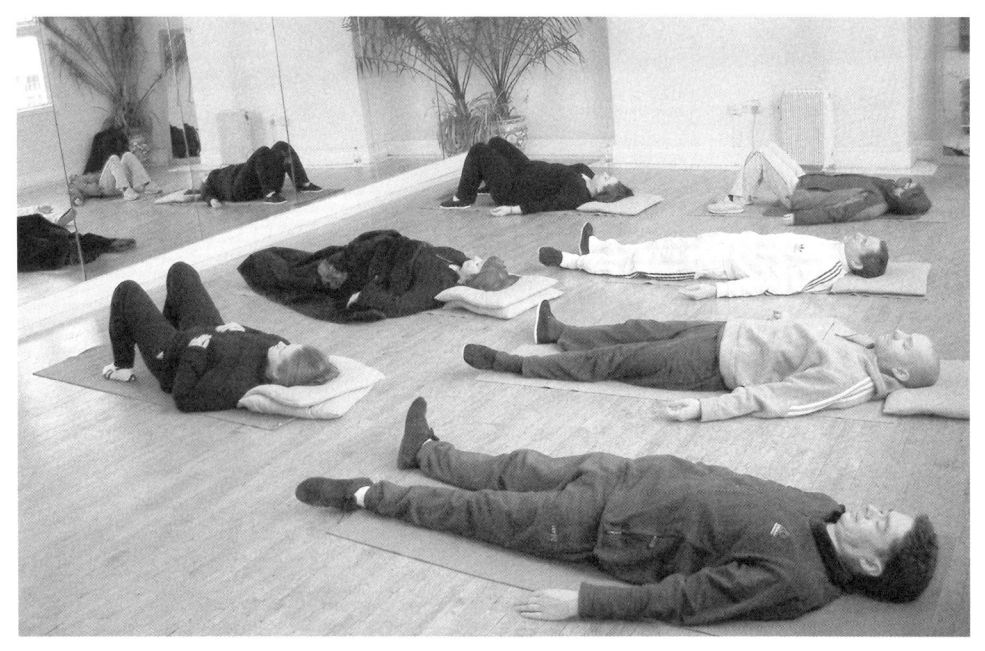

Relaxation exercises of this nature can be done for any length of time and as frequently as you like. The relaxation you develop in these sessions will help you in your everyday activities.

Chi Kung Practice

Chi Kung exercises are easy to do, they are not too complicated to remember. As relaxation is developed, energy is encouraged to flow. With the development of energy, more of it will flow to weaker, injured areas thus facilitating and increasing rejuvenation and healing. Increased relaxation will encourage more comfort in your practice.

When practising Chi Kung certain points need to be borne in mind.

- It is important to practise daily.
- Anyone can practice Chi Kung.
- It is possible to practise some of the exercises sitting or lying down which can be beneficial for specific physical conditions.
- Chi Kung can also work well with other forms of therapy.

The exercises illustrated are the ones that I feel can be learned from a book without necessarily having the guidance of a teacher. Tuition from a trained teacher is always preferable.

Chi Kung Exercises

Moving exercise

Exercise 1 - for gently stimulating and building the energy

Stand with your feet parallel, shoulder width apart, knees bent, arms resting by your sides. Throughout all the Chi Kung exercises the knees are kept bent. Have your tongue touching the roof of your mouth as if saying 'L' (do this throughout all the Chi Kung exercises).

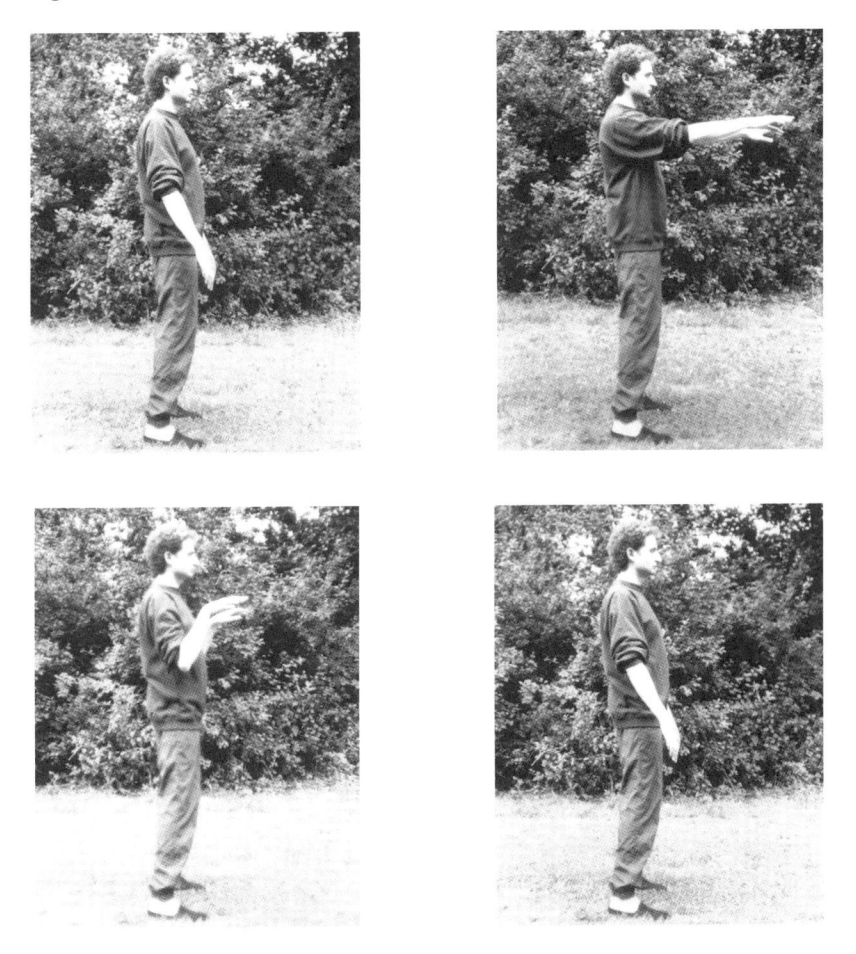

Slowly let your arms come up from the wrists up to shoulder height, slowly bring the fingers up as your hands come back towards your shoulders, as the elbows go down. Bring your hands down to your sides as if pushing down in water. Repeat the exercise imagining that you are moving in water. Once you have the hang of the movement, slow the speed down even more.

This sequence can be repeated for as long as you choose. Once familiar with the movement, co-ordinated breathing can be incorporated into the exercise Breathe in as the arms come up and the hands come towards the shoulders, breathe out as the hands go down. Allow the in and out breaths to be of similar lengths. Repeat this process. Make sure your back is straight and that you do not lean from side to side.

There are two opinions about breathing when practising moving Chi Kung. One is to have the breath follow the speed of the movement; the other is to allow the movement to follow the speed of the breath. Both need to work together. You can experiment with both ideas and choose which one suits you best.

Standing exercise

Exercise 2 - for concentrating the energy

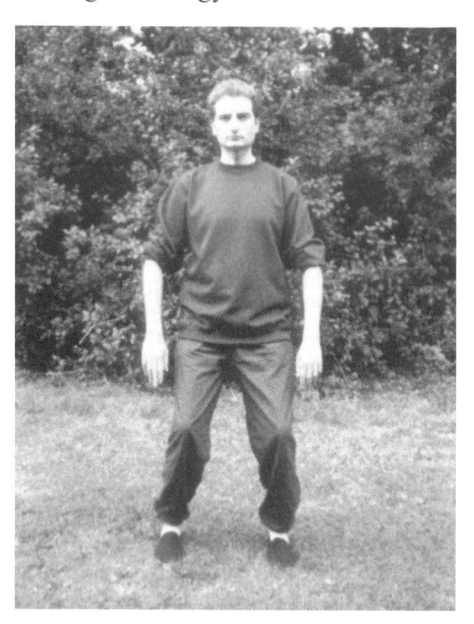

Stand feet parallel, shoulder width apart, heels in line, knees slightly bent. Have the tongue lightly touching the roof of your mouth. Arms are by your sides, slightly forward of the body, hands and fingers open, elbows slightly bent. Stay in this posture for as long as is comfortable, allowing the muscles to relax to help maintain the posture. To finish this exercise, come up in height and let your legs and arms relax. Repeat again if you desire. As your strength and stamina develop, you will be able to hold the posture for longer periods. It is important to keep your mind quiet and your body relaxed as you stand. Allow your breathing to take care of itself. The length of time spent standing like this can range from 2-10 minutes.

Moving Exercise

Exercise 3 - for circulating the energy

Repeat exercise 1 without focusing on the breath.

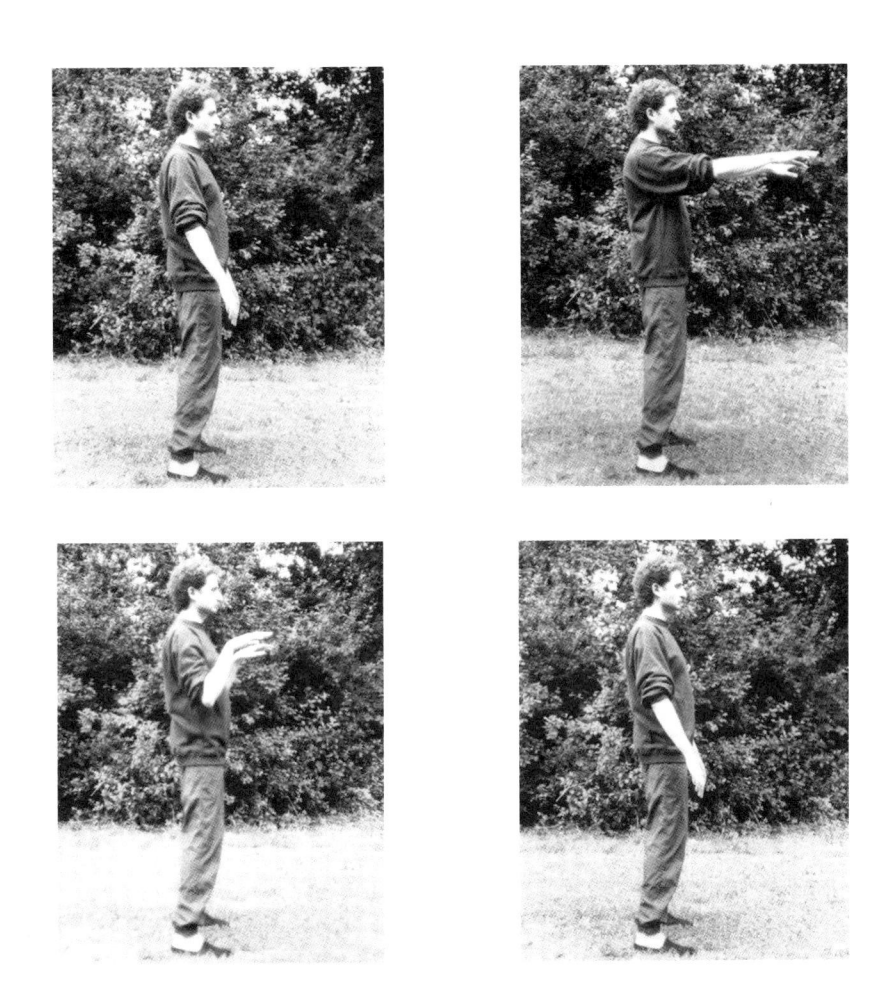

T'ai Chi Standing Postures

Some people believe that the benefits in T'ai chi come from the continuity of the movements, as one slowly passes from and through each posture to the next. Cheng Man-Ch'ing recommended that there be a smooth transition from one posture to the next, otherwise the flow of energy would be disrupted. He advocated the idea of moving as if in water so as to maintain evenness and relaxation. Stopping within the form was not encouraged so as not to interfere with continuity. In his classes, as with my own training, a large part of the lessons would involve having to stand in T'ai chi postures for an extended period of time, as the individual students in the class were each corrected on their postures.

It is acknowledged that standing in postures for elongated periods of time develops strength, endurance and increased capacity. Muscle exhaustion is also encouraged which leads to deeper levels of relaxation which the Chinese call 'sung'. In Cheng Man-Ch'ing T'ai chi this form of relaxation is advocated and encouraged. Out of this relaxation comes a feeling of weightedness as the weight of the body sinks into the ground. One has to let go in order to maintain the postures. Traditionally trained martial artists all undergo this form of standing training, not only to develop strength and character, but also power, which can then be expressed in their techniques.

Some people are of the opinion that too much concentration on practising standing postures can lead to stiffness in the execution of the moving forms, as the practitioners become attached to the feeling of fullness and solidity. It could be concluded that a combination of moving forms and static postures would bear most fruit and create a more all round practitioner.

We will now look at some static postures which can be practised separately or in conjunction with one's T'ai chi form practice.

Holding the Barrel

Most martial art systems have some variation of this posture.

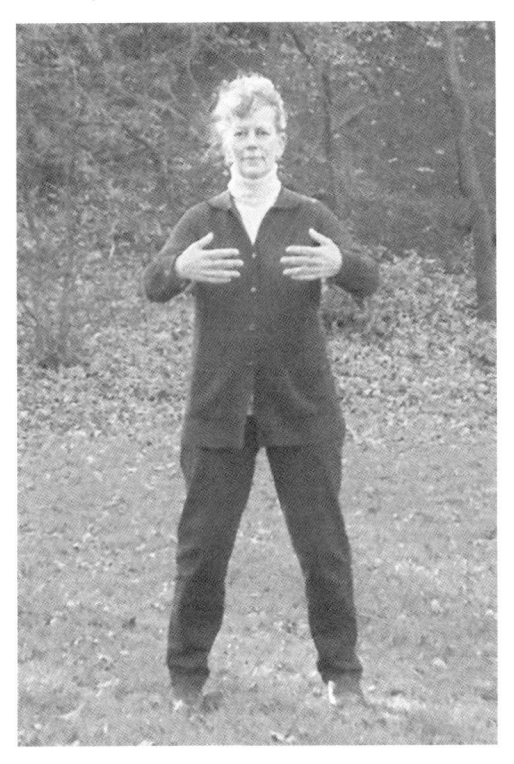

Stand with your feet parallel, shoulder width apart and in line. Bend the knees. Have the tongue touching the roof of the mouth. Bring your arms up and out in front of your chest with the middle fingers of each hand as if pointing towards each other. Imagine space underneath each armpit. Keep your shoulders down and relaxed. All you have to do is just stay in this posture, allowing your mind to be quiet and peaceful and allowing your body to be relaxed.

As time passes, the exercise becomes harder due to the fact that you are not moving. Your muscles will be working hard to maintain the posture, gravity will be making your arms even heavier. You will feel increasing demands on the arms, shoulders and thighs. The demand will turn to mild discomfort and then a feeling of burning as increased circulation is being pumped to those areas to deal with the demand. In order to maintain the posture you need to mentally focus on relaxing specific parts of the body. Maintaining the posture will make you stronger; the relaxation will help you maintain the posture. The exercise within itself will encourage you to develop relaxed strength.

The question is - how long do you hold the posture? This depends on your capacity, your objective and your tolerance for discomfort. It is acknowledged that lesser demand is good for health, greater demand is good for fitness and strength. Cheng Man-Ch'ing implied that if you are doing your training effectively then you will feel discomfort in your limbs.

It is important before adopting any rigorous physical exercise regime to either seek medical advice or be sure in yourself that you are up to the task.

It is recommended that after any long period of time spent practising static postures, you then do some form of slow moving sequence, whether it be T'ai chi or Chi Kung, so as to ensure that the energy is circulating and not pooled in certain areas of your body.

Once you have developed capacity to do this exercise for at least ten minutes at a time without coming up, you can then experiment with a wider foot stance of shoulder width and a half (this is known as Chinese horse stance). This stance, due to the width, means that your torso is lower down and your thighs will be working even harder. Over time your body will adapt to most demands. The important thing is not to rush your progress and not push your body too much, too soon.

Holding the barrel posture is seen as essential training in most T'ai chi styles, otherwise the practitioner will not have a good foundation, as well as what is called 'root'. Root is the ability to be solid on the ground so that you are not easily pushed.

Relaxing, sinking and being rooted are important aspects of the Cheng Man-Ch'ing T'ai chi tradition.

Play Guitar

In the Cheng Man-Ch'ing system, play guitar is probably one of the most important exercises to practise. Cheng recommended his students spend time practising this posture. He stated that by doing this exercise certain meridians in the body would be opened so as to encourage increased flow of energy through them. As the students became stronger, Cheng would recommend that they sink and sit even lower on the back leg. This training will encourage greater potential mobility in the solo T'ai chi form performance. More importantly it will develop the yin (soft) aspect of T'ai chi. Some styles of T'ai chi are known for the yang (full/hard) aspect of their techniques. Cheng's style is known for its softness. This aspect is important, for the health development nature is within the yin (softness), as energy will be encouraged to flow freely through the body.

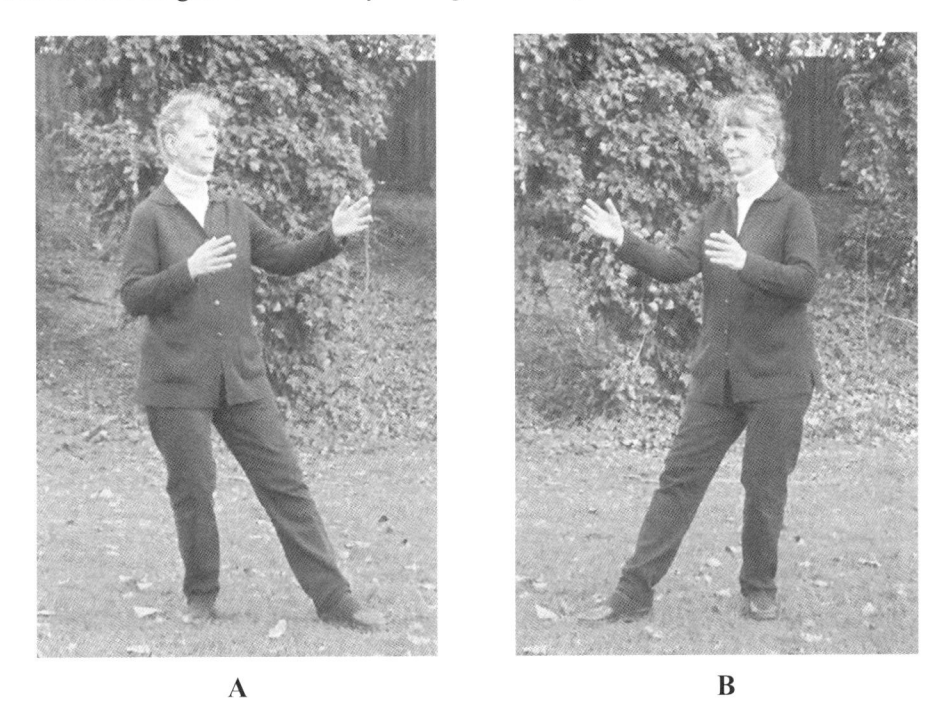

A   B

(A) Turn the right toes out, as if to the corner of a room, bend both knees. Move all the weight onto the right leg, bring the left leg forward and rest the left foot on the floor but without placing any weight onto it.

Raise both arms as if playing a guitar. Left hand extended further than the right. Right palm is facing left elbow, with comfortable space underneath your armpits.

This posture will be harder to maintain than holding the barrel as all the weight is on one leg and one thigh will be working much harder.

Initially hold the posture until you feel the legs beginning to work then come up and relax. Repeat on the other side which is referred to as mirror image.**(B)**

It is advisable to do the exercise for an equal length of time on each side. One way to achieve this is by watching the second hand of a clock.

Start perhaps for 30 seconds each side, increasing slowly to a minute, and with consistent practice you will be able to maintain longer periods of time. Do not push yourself too much too soon because you want to maintain your enthusiasm - this could be influenced by too much discomfort too often.

Single Whip

This posture was recommended by Cheng Man-Ch'ing as a way of developing the yang aspect of T'ai chi as it has a stronger feel to it. It is also good for the lungs as you are exercising the muscles in the chest and back.

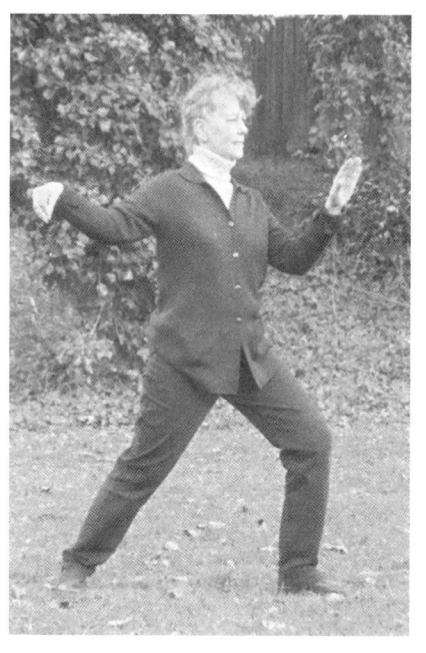

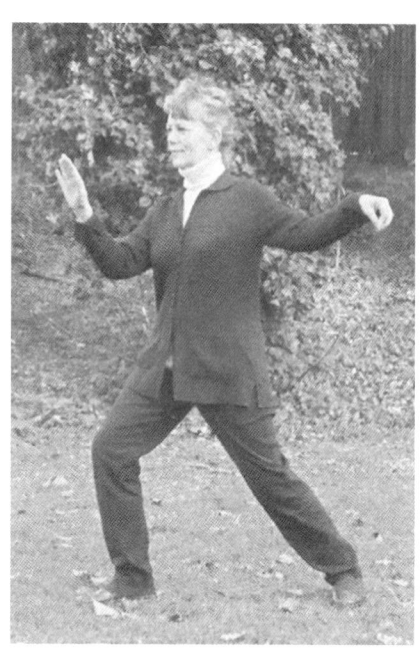

A   B

(A) Stand feet parallel, shoulder width. Turn the right toes out at an angle of 45 degrees to the left foot. Bend the knees and transfer all the weight onto the right foot. Step forward with the left foot maintaining shoulder width between the heels. Shift the weight onto the left foot so that there is 70 % of your weight on the left foot and 30 % on the right. Lift your right hand up and make a beak shape, bending at the wrist, all the tips of the fingers meeting the tip of the thumb. The top of the beak needs to be shoulder height and the beak is extended out from your shoulder so that the arm is extended but not locked. Raise the left hand to chest height and extend forward without bending at the wrist too much. Stay in this posture. Tongue touching the roof of the mouth. The main demand will be felt in the front leg, especially the thigh.

When you feel you have to come up, come up slowly, bringing your feet closer together, do not fidget and allow your body to recover naturally. Observe how you feel, this will give you feedback on the effect of the exercise.

Continue by doing mirror image of this posture.**(B)**

Using a clock will make sure that you spend equal time on both versions. Over time your ability to stay in the postures for longer periods will develop. Any of the other postures in the T'ai chi form can be held, as well as done mirror image. With consistent practice over time your stamina, endurance and strength will develop and improve. The static postures practised in conjunction with the T'ai chi form will give you all round benefit and development.

Ponder This

Exercise your body, empty your mind, only think when you have to and the rest of the time enjoy yourself.

How many people exercise their bodies? When do they have the time? Work and family commitments, amongst other things, take up most of their time. How many people empty their minds? We amass information; we are encouraged to think constantly. We entertain our minds with TV, films, videos, radio etc. We seldom slow down our thought process. How many people really enjoy themselves and have fun? Some say they do but often only through artificial means (alcohol, drugs). Our search for peace of mind is often from outside, from some external form, human or artificial. We have lost the ability to look inwards for our own happiness and satisfaction.

Let's look at this saying more closely: *'Exercise your body, empty your mind, only think when you have to and the rest of the time enjoy yourself.'*

1. Exercise your body. Many people find it difficult to empty their minds of thoughts. Those who practise meditation comment on how difficult this task is. The mind by its nature wants to be active. One way to achieve this stillness of mind is to be involved in some form of physical activity. Doing something physical involves concentration. This fact alone brings attention and mental focus to the activity. Over time, doing a simple physical activity can bring the mind to an even calmer, quieter place. Let us also not forget the physiological benefits of exercising.

2. Empty your mind. Emptying the mind of thoughts can lead one to a place of peace and calm. One's perception may become clearer as there are less clouding thoughts to obscure the scenery. This mental state can lead to the experience of being in the moment. (Some authorities say this is the function of meditation - to be in the moment. It means you are totally focused on the task at hand).

3. Only think when you have to. Thinking is something we do but is it necessary all the time? The ability to think is useful, so is the ability to not think. Our mind is generally full of thoughts. The Chinese call the mind the 'monkey' because it is always chattering. They recommend that we empty the mind at times as a way of achieving balance.

4. The rest of the time enjoy yourself. Enjoyment is a state of mind. Ask a person in the street if they are happy. They may answer yes, no or relatively. Many people's inner state of happiness is dependent on the external situation being correct in relation to their desires. This is often not the case and may lead to unhappiness. Unhappiness generally occurs because people have expectations to begin with of what they want, or what they think they should have. If these are not met, unhappiness is often the result.

Applying these above ideas may improve the quality of life. There is one way to find out! If through practising T'ai chi, Chi Kung and meditation we can minimise and remove thoughts of a negative, distracting nature then the thoughts we do have will have more potential to be effective. All of this will heighten the probability of our creating the life we want for ourselves.

SECTION THREE

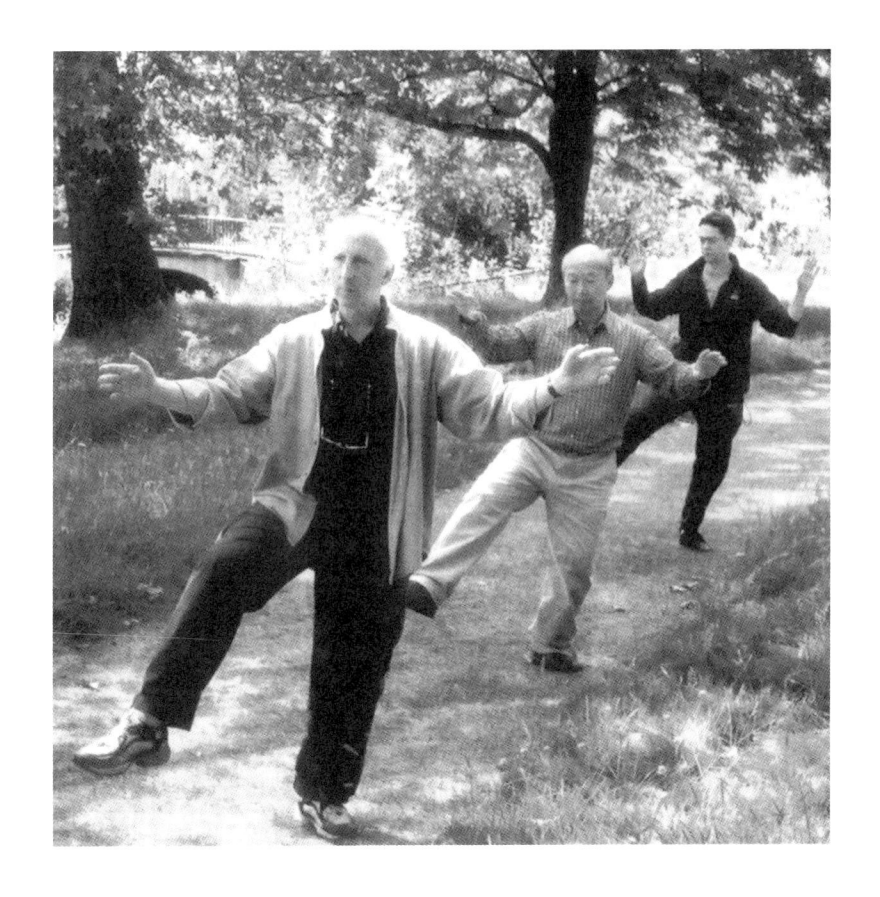

T'ai Chi Ch'uan - the benefits

As we have seen the Taoist art of T'ai Chi Ch'uan (commonly referred to as T'ai chi) was originally developed as a form of martial art, but over the years the emphasis has centered more on health than fighting. The T'ai chi form is characterised by its slow, even movements. These movements exercise every important joint in the body. When practised regularly T'ai chi helps the body's ability to resist illness, to adapt to the external environment and to restore proper internal functioning. Anyone can maintain a reasonable level of fitness through practising T'ai chi.

The healing qualities of T'ai chi have been well documented over the centuries. Even the 20th century's most renowned and respected Grandmaster, Professor Cheng Man-Ch'ing started the practice of T'ai chi as a result of ill health. T'ai chi, by its nature, is an ideal health exercise as it is moderate and slow. Some very strenuous activities can leave one feeling high and exhilarated, sometimes followed by exhaustion. In those cases the body has borrowed from its reserves of energy. T'ai chi, on the other hand, is always replenishing the body's reserves.

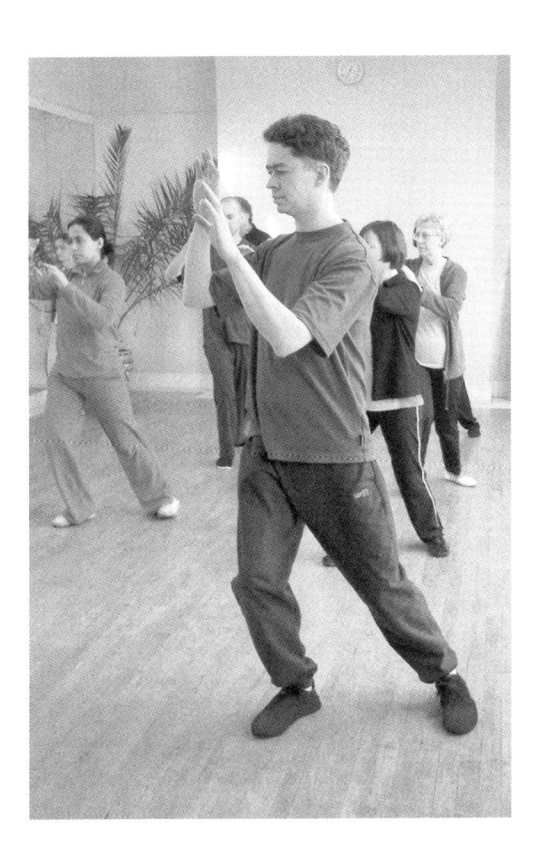

The low postures included in the T'ai chi form increase the body's demand and consumption of oxygen. Oxygen plays an important positive part in protecting the body from age related deterioration. The lower your oxygen consumption, the less vitality you will have, reducing your resistance to illness. A unique feature of T'ai chi is that it promotes mental as well as physical relaxation; it is often described as a form of moving meditation.

It has been confirmed through clinical studies in China that there is a connection between the practice of T'ai Chi Ch'uan and lower blood pressure. A Peking study compared two groups of over-50 year olds and found that the group which did T'ai chi had substantially lower blood pressure due to muscle relaxation, which helped establish a conditioned relaxation in the blood vessels, which lowered blood pressure. This relaxation also helps people with high blood pressure by countering over activity in the cerebral cortex and vasomotor centre which regulates the size of blood vessels and may cause blood pressure to rise.

While performing the T'ai chi form emphasis is placed not on the breathing, but on the form; the low postures naturally increase the body's demand for oxygen. T'ai chi, if properly done, can improve blood supply to the muscles and to the connective tissues surrounding the joints, resulting in an improvement in the metabolic process in the cartilage, bone and muscle. Consistent practice makes joints more flexible and ligaments more elastic. Muscular strength is also increased.

The late Professor Cheng Man-Ch'ing considered health to be a prerequisite to anything else. He wrote, 'If one possesses only talent, without considering physical health as a worthy supplement, then what will be the outcome?' He believed that one's physical health should be equal to one's mental as well as physical talents.

Learning

There are basically three ways to learn a physical skill:

1. From example
2. From verbal instruction
3. From physical correction

This section of the book will give visual images to follow as well as written instruction. Nothing can replace tuition with a competent teacher. It is highly recommended that if at all possible you attend classes. The advantages are consolidation of personal practice, following advice and guidance from a teacher, as well as the benefits of practising with a group.

The traditional way of learning T'ai chi is to learn one posture at a time, only moving on to the next posture when the previous one has been mastered. This process is repeated to the end of the form. I recommend this way of learning.

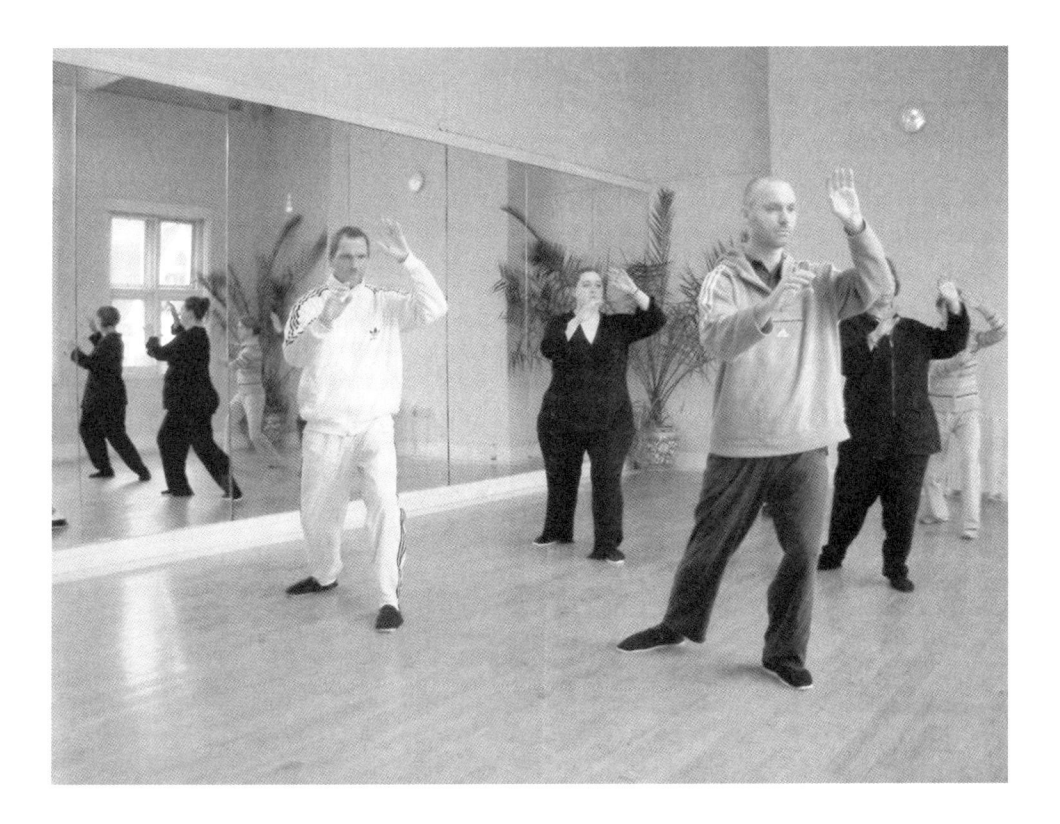

GUIDELINES FOR SUCCESSFUL T'AI CHI CH'UAN PRACTICE

Success in learning any skill, including T'ai chi, is dependent on three criteria: good tuition and example, learner's level of natural ability, personal practice.

With correct tuition progress can be much faster as there is less opportunity for error. Rhythm and pace of learning, and capacity for acquiring new information determines the speed of progress. Success in learning T'ai chi depends to a large extent on practice. More specifically: the quality of practice, the quantity of practice, the purpose of practice.

Quality of Practice

The quality of any practice depends on total focus, preventing distraction from external stimuli or thoughts. The intricate T'ai chi movements ensure your focus will be engaged, reducing the mind's inclination to wander. All your mental focus will be taken up with executing the movements accurately.

Quantity of Practice

Developing a skill requires practice. Time has to be spent repeating movements to a point where no conscious thought is needed. To get to this point hours of consistent, conscientious, correct practice will have had to be undertaken. Your physical condition and natural aptitude for T'ai chi will dictate just how many hours will be required. The more you practise in a concentrated period of time the further you can go; short bursts of practice at irregular intervals will not work so well.

Practising can be compared to rowing a boat up a river against the current. Cease rowing and you will go backwards, therefore you must constantly row (practise) to make progress.

If you find yourself engaged in mindless practice stop. Shorter amounts of quality practice will better help you improve your T'ai chi studies.

Purpose of Practice

The primary aim of practice is to improve in whatever skill you choose. However, depending on the state and level of your focus and intention, one of three things can happen: improvement, stagnation, or deterioration.

Without intention you can quite easily go backwards in your level of ability. Some people become complacent, satisfied by their current state of proficiency and will only practise to remain at that level. To progress a decision to improve will be necessary as well as to the extent of that improvement.

Demand

To improve mentally or physically you need to give yourself a demand that exceeds your current capacity. Your mind and body will adapt appropriately to meet that added demand thereby increasing your capacity to meet other, possibly greater demands. Once you have gone beyond what you perceived as your limit you will realise you can do much more than you thought possible.

Goals and Deadlines

Goals and deadlines will help you organise your actions around what you want. Growth occurs as a result of movement towards goals. Having a place to go will focus your actions. By setting challenging and ever increasing goals as a form of motivation to improve, you will progress faster and better maximise the use of your time.

Training

Get into the habit of setting aside specific times every day for your practice, in that way it will be easier to maintain progress. T'ai chi can be practised at any time of day, the most beneficial times being first thing in the morning and last thing at night. It is preferable not to practise just before, nor immediately after eating. You can practise as often and for as long as you wish. Remember you can achieve a high level of proficiency irrespective of your talent and ability.

When learning something new there is often enthusiasm and excitement, however after a period of time you may reach a point when little seems to be happening. In fact, assimilation and consolidation is occurring; your learning is becoming part of you. When you continue beyond this stage you begin to develop ability in your specific skill, which generates more enthusiasm and should encourage more practice.

Relaxation

The key to doing T'ai chi well is relaxation, without it your movements will be stiff and disjointed. The quality of your form practice will be improved as a result of reduced tension throughout the body.

Balance

An integral part of T'ai chi is physical balance - refer to 'Points to bear in mind'. Adherence to these principles will lead to improved co-ordination.

Mind

In order to relax the body one needs to clear the mind of distracting thoughts, allowing them to come and go without holding on to them. By concentrating on and being attentive to what you are doing, your mind becomes focused and calm.

The Influence of Thoughts

The way you think about yourself will influence your T'ai chi practice. Negative thoughts relating to your ability will slow down your progress. By quietening your mind and focusing on your movements you begin to silence these distracting thoughts. Once these are quiet you can consciously choose constructive thoughts which will help your progress. Often a different attitude of mind can make the difference between doing your T'ai chi well or badly.

Accuracy of Movement

It is important to remember to work on accuracy of movement. Incorrect practice is of little value in any activity. Remember: quality not quantity. Your time is much better spent doing a small amount well rather than a lot badly. Do not rush your progress. The use of a large mirror can help you correct your postures. With this book you are your own teacher. The responsibility for your practice, motivation and progress is yours alone.

Keeping your Motivation

An important aspect of learning anything is maintaining interest and motivation. To be able to keep that motivation going, give yourself sensible challenges along the way, challenges that will demand your attention and interest. Following along with this book gives you an opportunity to be totally in charge of your actions and progress.

Enjoyment and Pleasure

It is worth remembering that anything done with pleasure has more energy and enjoyment.

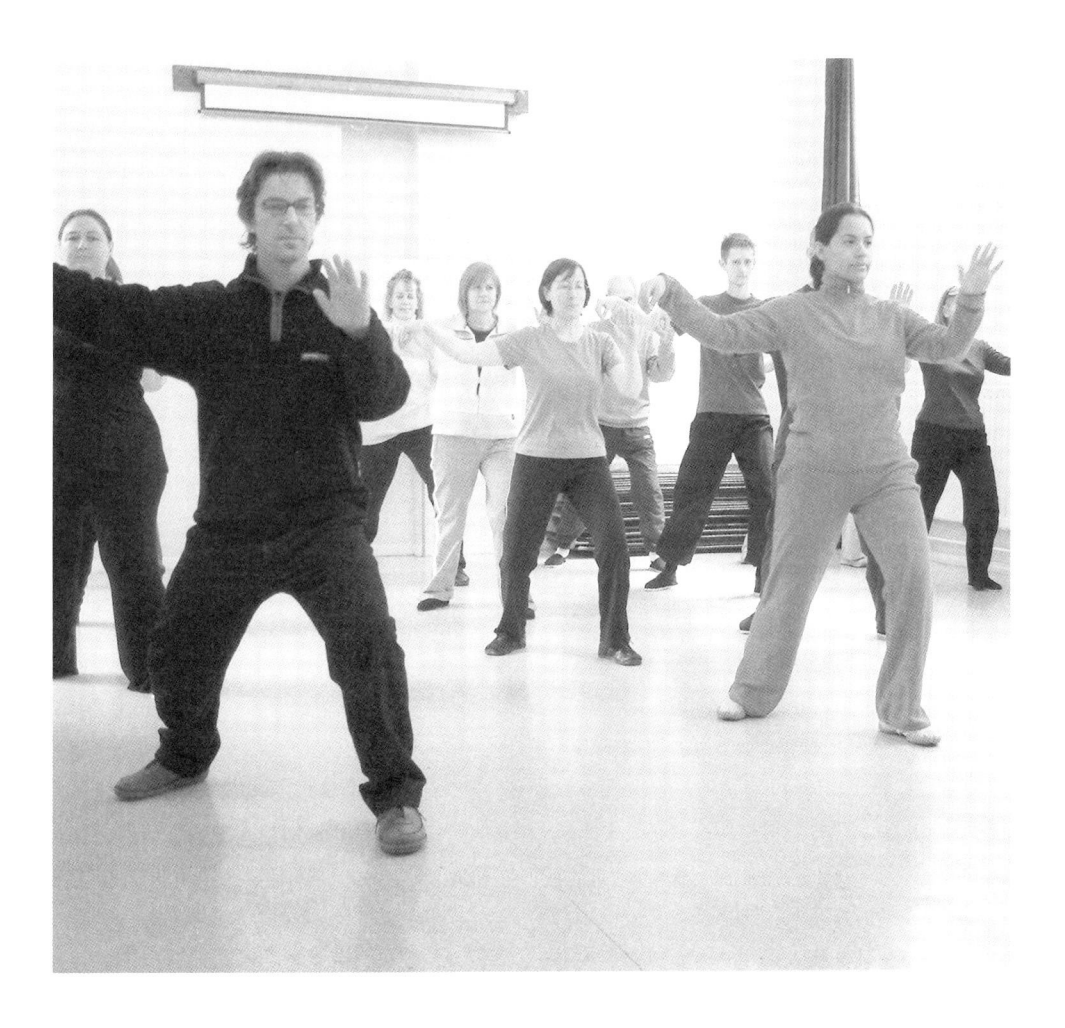

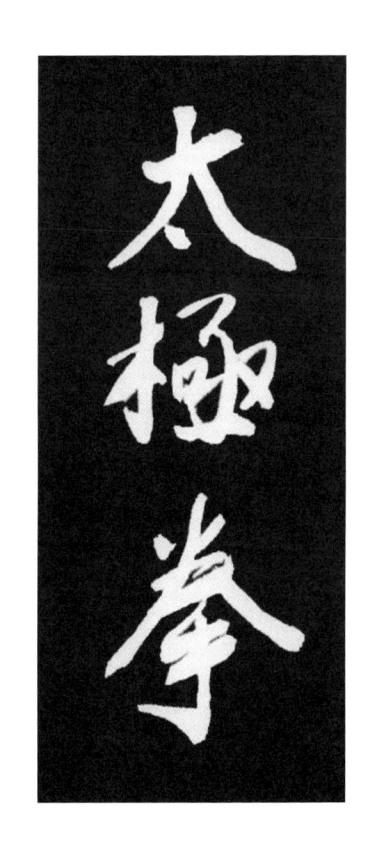

CHENG MAN-CH'ING SHORT FORM

太極拳

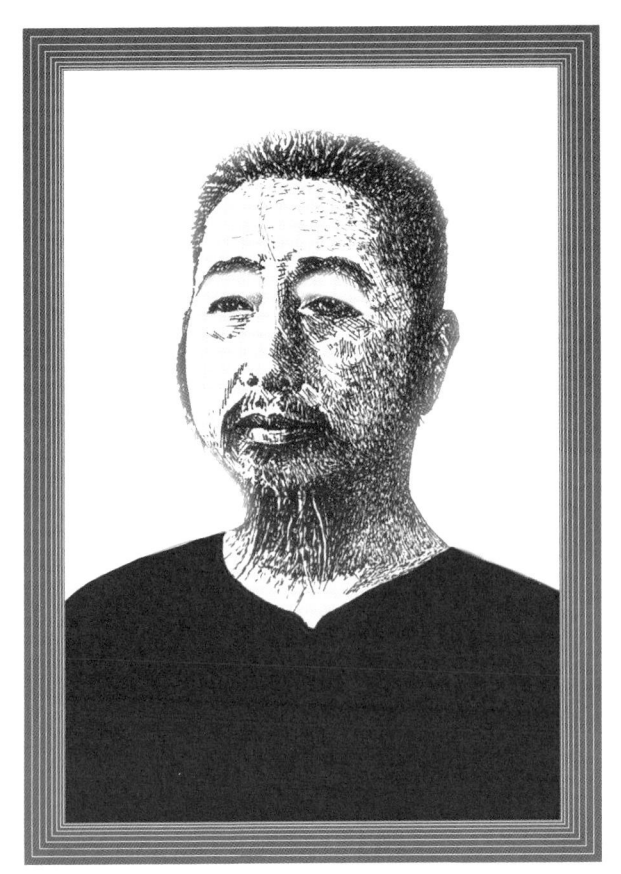

Cheng Man-Ch'ing

Professor Cheng Man-Ch'ing was born in the Chekiang Province of China in 1901. He died in T'aipei, Taiwan in 1975. He taught T'ai chi in China, Taiwan and America. His own study of T'ai chi started as a result of ill health, having developed tuberculosis in his 20's.

He studied the Yang long T'ai chi form with Yang Cheng-fu, a famous T'ai chi Master, who was a direct descendent of the Yang family. Professor Cheng at a later date shortened the Yang form by nearly two thirds to 37 postures for ease of practice. While reducing the number of postures he still maintained the essential elements.

The Professor's writing and teaching have been influential in promoting T'ai chi in the West. He was a man of many talents. As well as being a T'ai chi Master he was also an accomplished painter, calligrapher, poet and practitioner of Traditional Chinese Medicine.

SHORT FORM - Posture Names

PART ONE

Preparation

Beginning

Grasp the Sparrow's Tail Ward Off Left

Grasp the Sparrow's Tail Ward Off Right

Grasp the Sparrow's Tail Roll Back

Grasp the Sparrow's Tail Press

Grasp the Sparrow's Tail Push

Single Whip

Play Guitar/Play the Pipa

Lean Forward

White Crane Spreads Wings

Brush Left Knee and Twist Step

Play Guitar

Brush Left Knee and Twist Step

Step Forward, Deflect Downward, Intercept and Punch

Withdraw and Push

Crossing Hands

PART TWO

Embrace the Tiger to Return to the Mountain

Grasp the Sparrow's Tail Roll Back

Grasp the Sparrow's Tail Press

Grasp the Sparrow's Tail Push

Single Whip Facing the Corner

Fist Under Elbow

Repulse Monkey (Right and Left)

Diagonal Flying

Wave Hands in the Clouds

Single Whip

Snake Creeps Down (Squat Single Whip)

Golden Cockerel Stands on Left Leg

Golden Cockerel Stands on Right Leg

Separate the Right Foot

Separate the Left Foot

Turn Around and Strike with Heel

Brush Left Knee

Brush Right Knee

Step Forward and Strike with Fist

Step Forward and Ward off Right

Grasp the Sparrow's Tail Roll Back

Grasp the Sparrow's Tail Press

Grasp the Sparrow's Tail Push

Single Whip

PART TWO continued

Fair Lady Weaving with her Shuttle

Grasp the Sparrow's Tail Ward Off Left

Grasp the Sparrow's Tail Ward Off Right

Grasp the Sparrow's Tail Roll Back

Grasp the Sparrow's Tail Press

Grasp the Sparrow's Tail Push

Single Whip

Snake Creeps Down (Squat Single Whip)

Step Forwards to the Seven Stars of the Dipper

Step Back to Ride the Tiger

Turn Body and Sweep Lotus with Leg (Lotus Kick)

Bend the Bow to Shoot the Tiger

Step Forward , Deflect Down, Intercept and Punch

Withdraw and Push

Crossing Hands

Conclusion

POINTS TO BEAR IN MIND

- The head is always held erect as if suspended from above
- The back is straight
- The pelvic bone is slightly tucked under to help straighten the lower back
- Shoulders relaxed, hanging down naturally
- Chest relaxed
- Keep the elbows down
- The knee does not go over the front toes
- Movement is initiated from the hips
- The legs are relaxed
- At the end of a posture the hips are straight
- Focus your mind in the tan tien, an area approximately two inches below the navel
- Allow the breathing to be relaxed
- The tongue touches the roof of the mouth
- Movements are smooth and even
- Allow the mind to be calm and quiet
- Consistent practice is essential for progress

INSTRUCTIONS FOR LEARNING THE FORM

Stand upright, heels together, toes apart. Imagine your head is suspended from above and a weight pulling your coccyx down, tuck pelvic bone under slightly, this will help to straighten your lower back, shoulders relaxed, tongue touching the roof of your mouth.

PREPARATION

Sink all your weight into the right leg as you bend your knees. Hands come into the ready position. Lift left foot to the side, shoulder width heel first, toes straight. Shift weight into the left foot, turn hips to the right slightly, turn hips back straight, turn right toes in, parallel with left. Bring weight to centre, stand erect without locking your knees.

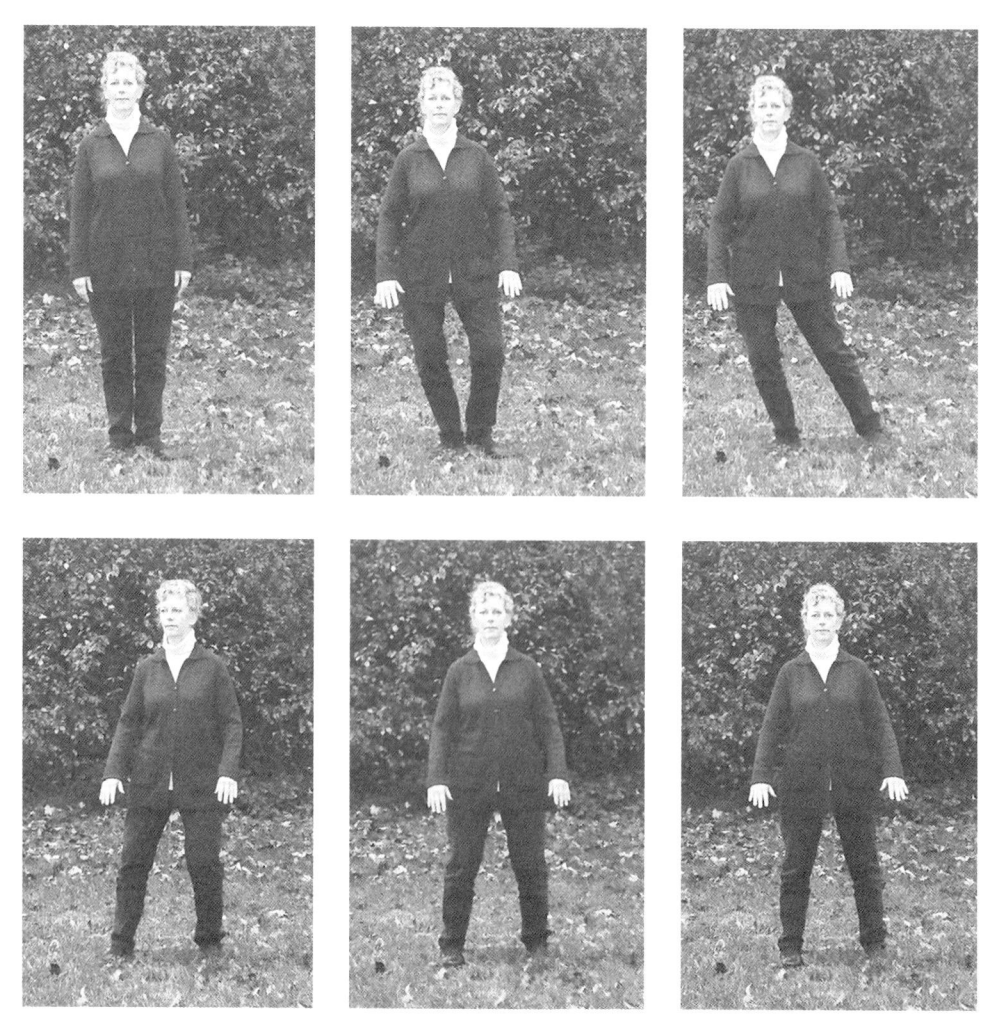

BEGINNING

Hands begin to rise as if being pulled up by the wrists, elbows remain bent. When wrists reach shoulder height the fingers open. Fingers relax as the hands come back towards your shoulders, as the elbows go down. Hands float down as if moving in water, then up to the ready position.

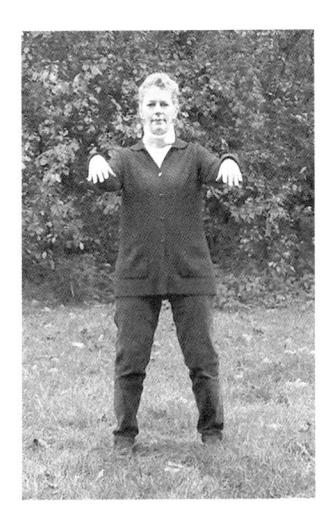

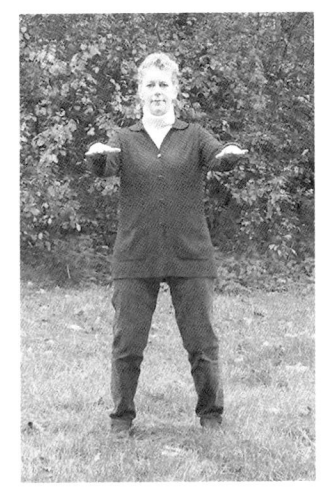

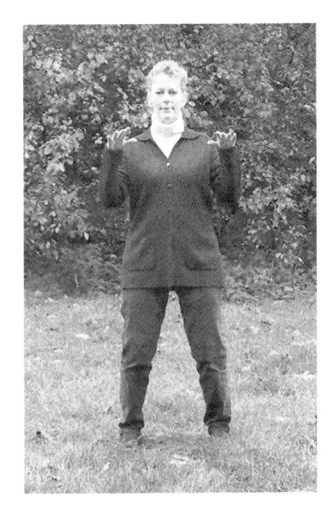

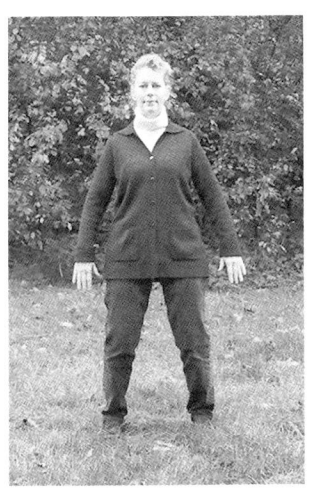

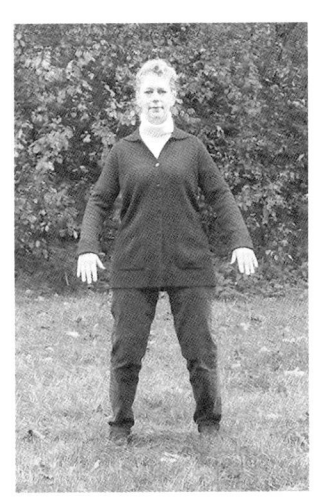

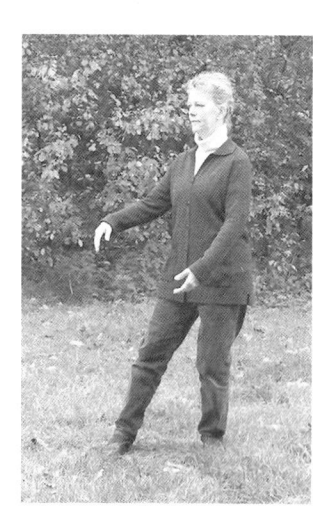

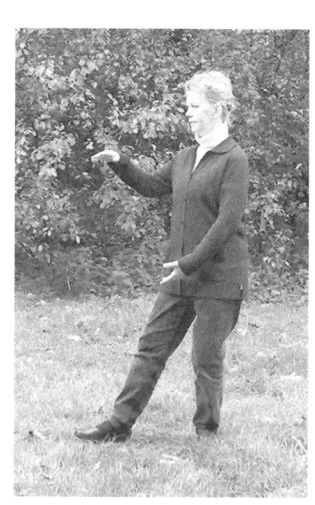

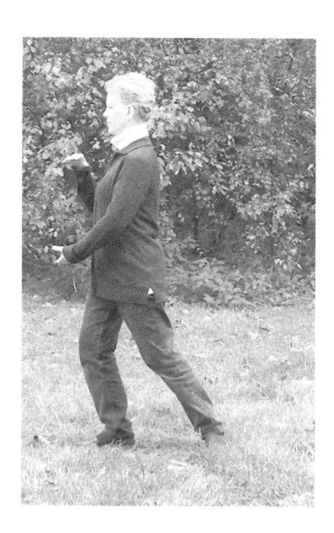

GRASP THE SPARROW'S TAIL WARD OFF LEFT

Sink all your weight into the left foot, pivot on the right heel toes pointing up, as the right hand rises and the left hand moves underneath. Step onto the right foot, both palms are facing each other as if holding a beach ball. You are now on the ball of your left foot. Step forward with the left foot onto the left heel keeping shoulder width between the heels, place the foot down, toes straight. As you shift into the left leg, left hand rises, right hand comes down. When over 50% of your weight is in the left foot turn the hips to straight, the right toes turn in at a 45° angle. The finished posture is left palm facing the chest, the right hand down by your right side in front. 70% of the weight is in the left leg, 30% in the right.

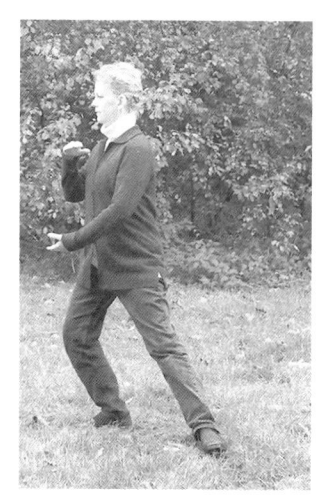

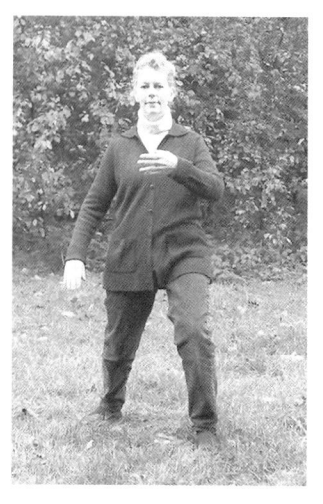

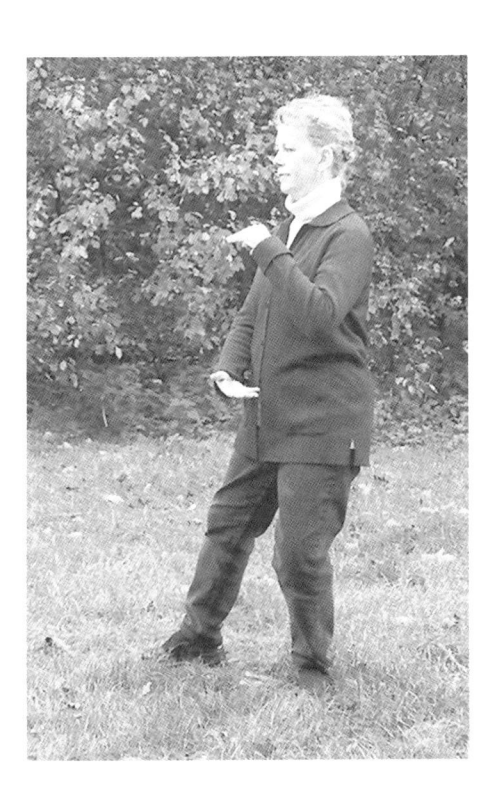

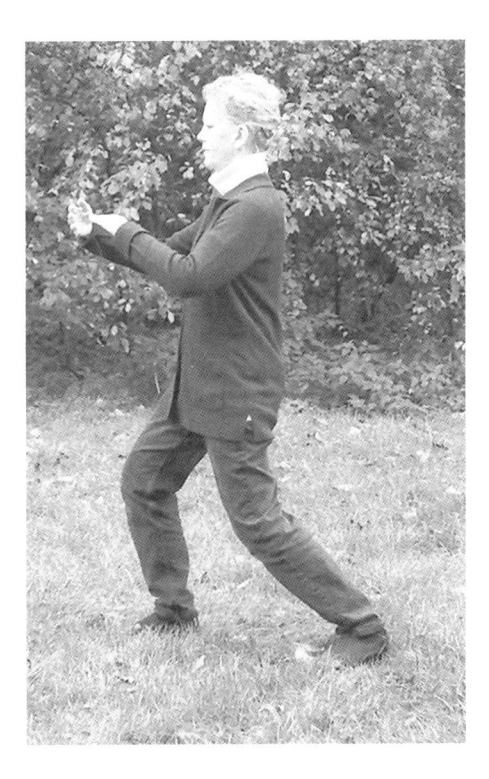

GRASP THE SPARROW'S TAIL WARD OFF RIGHT

Shift all the weight into the left foot as you turn on the ball of the right foot. Bring the right palm underneath the left, as if holding a beach ball. Step out widely onto the right heel. Shift weight into the right foot as the right hand rises to chest height, the left fingers pointing at right palm. Turn hips to the right facing east, the left toes turn in at a 45° angle, 70% of weight in front foot, body facing east.

GRASP THE SPARROW'S TAIL ROLL BACK

Turn your waist to the right 10°, keeping the weight distribution the same. Sit back onto your left leg. As you turn, the left hand comes down round and up in an arc of a circle to ear height, while the right hand comes in front of your body. All your weight is in your left foot.

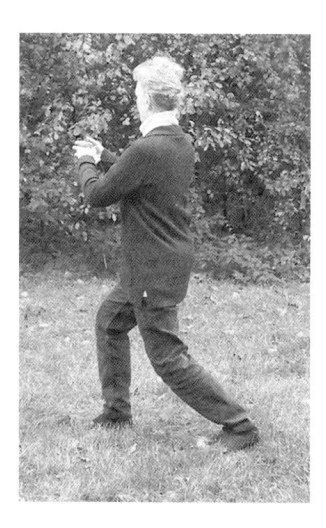

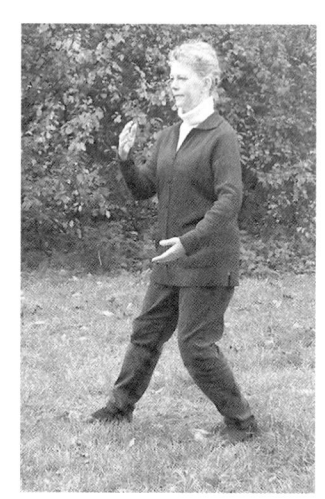

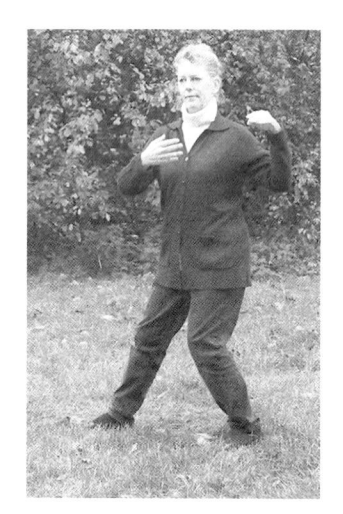

GRASP THE SPARROW'S TAIL PRESS

Shift weight back into the right foot as the left palm comes forward to touch the right inner wrist, chest height, hips straight. 70% of weight in right foot.

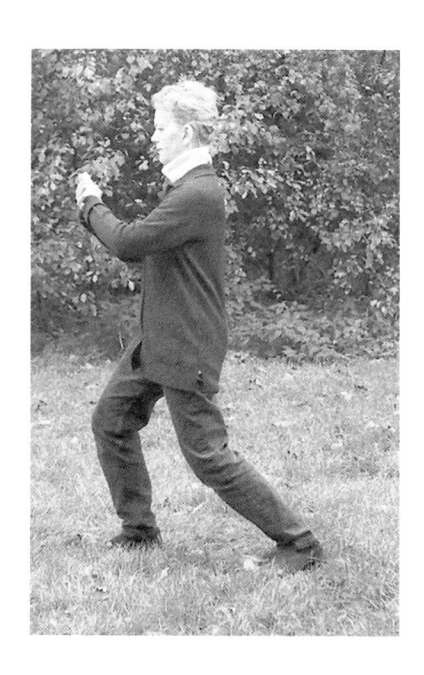

GRASP THE SPARROW'S TAIL PUSH

Sit back onto the left leg, hands separate, shift into your right leg, push with the hands, fingertips shoulder height and chest width, elbows bent. 70% of your weight on the front leg.

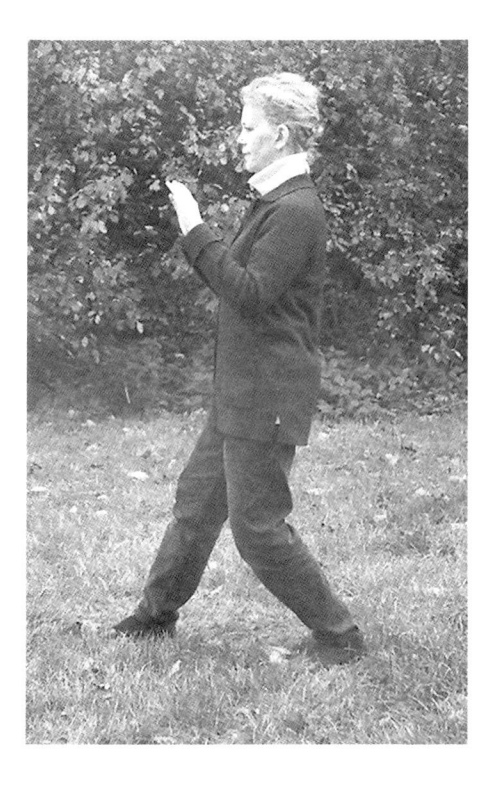

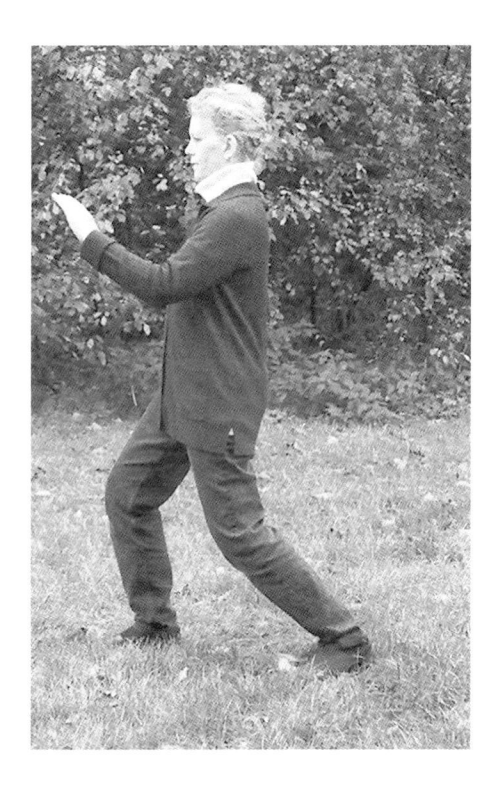

SINGLE WHIP

Sit back onto your left leg, the arms come down parallel to the ground, elbows slightly bent, all the weight is in your left leg. Turn your torso and the right toes to the left as far as they will go, your nose, navel and arms maintaining the same relationship to each other. Shift the weight back into the right foot as you turn the waist to the right. Left hand comes down with the palm facing up underneath the right hand, all the fingers of which are joined in the shape of a bird's beak. All the weight is on your right foot. Turn the hips to the left and pivot on the ball of the left foot, the right hand formed as a beak moves out to the corner, shoulder height. Step out widely onto your left heel. Shift the weight into the left foot, the left hand rises in front of you, turn your waist to the west, the right toes turn in at an angle of 45º, at the last moment the left palm turns over.

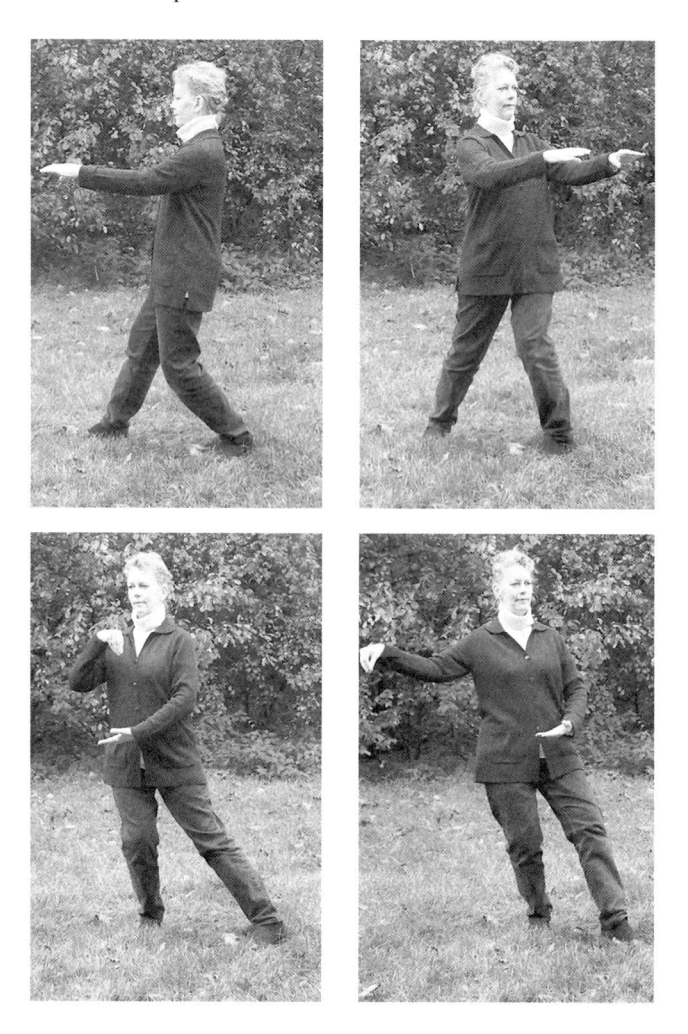

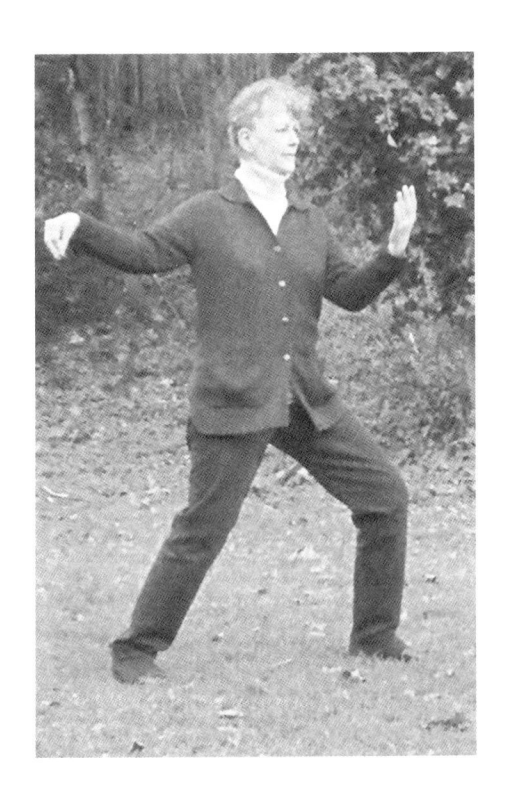

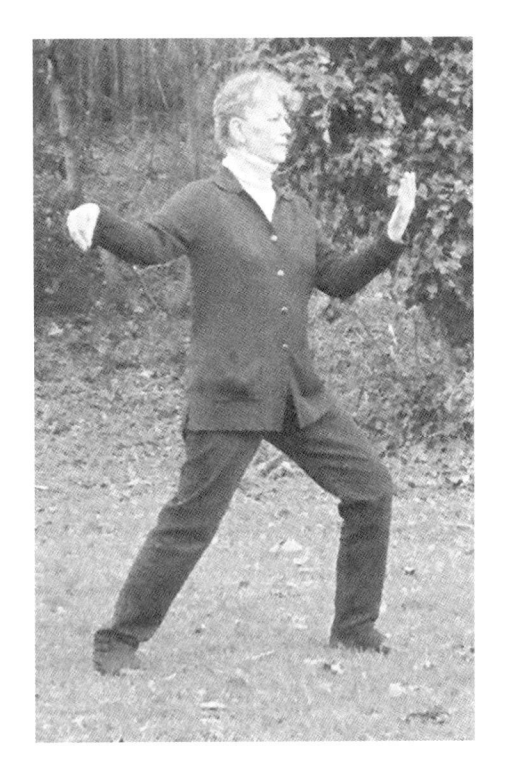

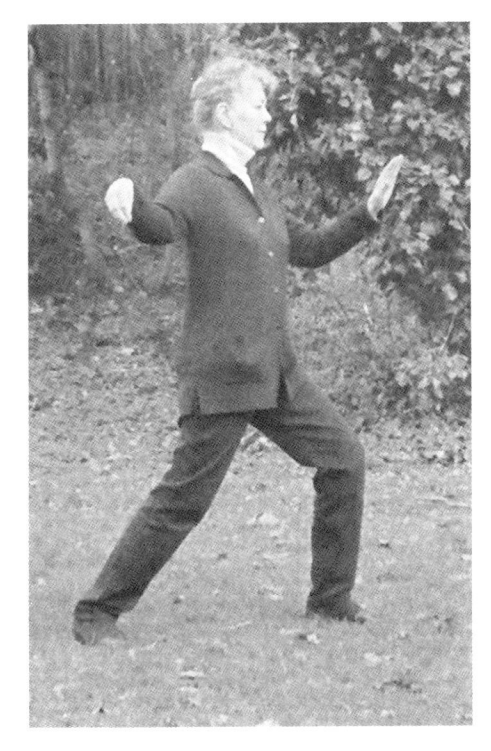

PLAY GUITAR/PLAY THE PIPA

Shift all the weight into the left foot, turn on the ball of the right foot, as you turn your waist 90° to the right. Arms face each other with the left palm facing the right elbow. Right heel comes into line with the left heel, right toes off the ground, as you bring the arms closer to each other. All your weight is in the left leg.

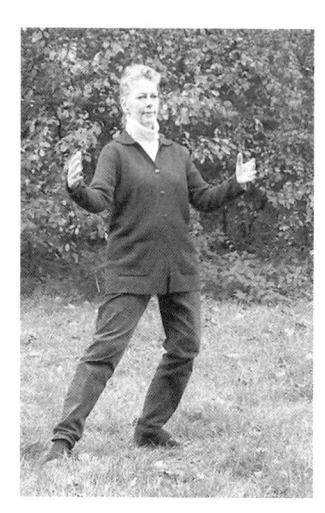

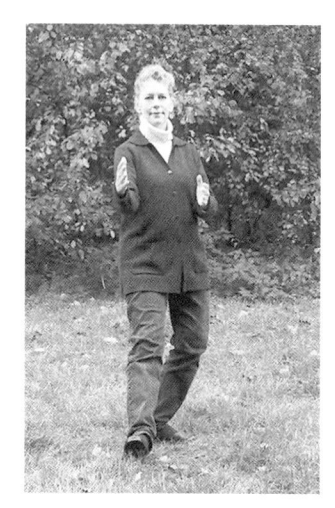

LEAN FORWARD

Right foot drops back towards left foot, hands come down, right palm protecting the groin, while left arm remains relaxed by left side, right foot resting on the ball. Step out onto the right foot, shift weight into right foot, lead into the movement with your shoulder, right elbow slightly bent, left palm by right elbow. 70% of weight in the right leg.

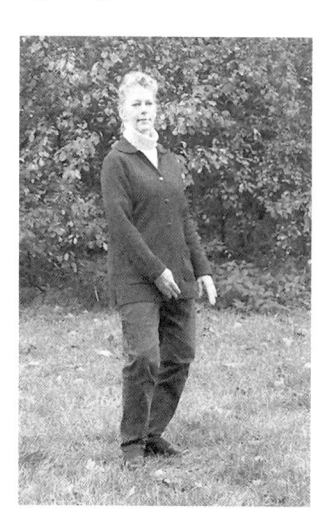

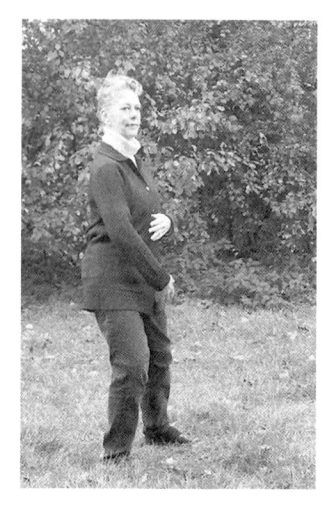

WHITE CRANE SPREADS WINGS

All the weight comes into the right foot. Simultaneously the left foot slides forward in line with the right resting on the ball as the right hand comes up to protect the right temple, the left hand brushes knee.

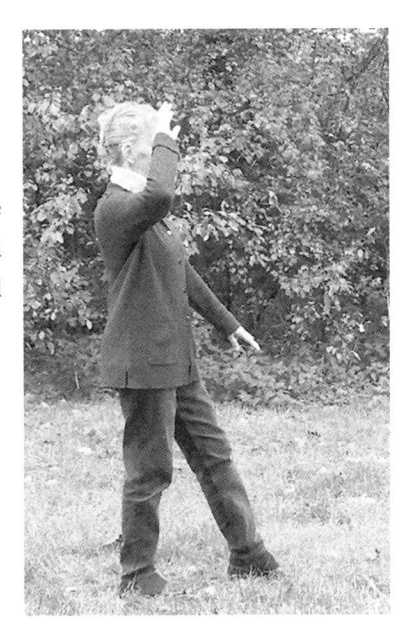

BRUSH LEFT KNEE AND TWIST STEP

Sink your weight into the right foot as you turn to the right turning on the ball of the left foot. Right hand moves down round and back in an arc of a circle up to the right ear, wrist relaxed, as the left hand comes up round and down. Step out widely onto your left foot, weight shifts into the left foot. Brush knee with left hand, strike with right, right toes turn in at 45°angle, 70% of weight in front foot, shoulder width between the heels, waist straight facing west.

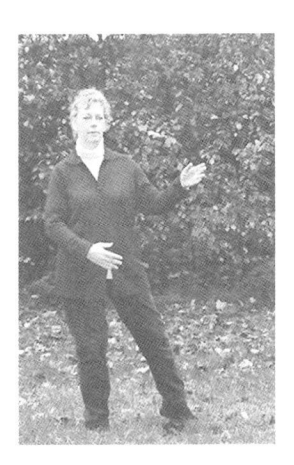

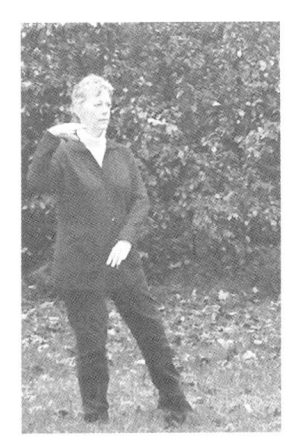

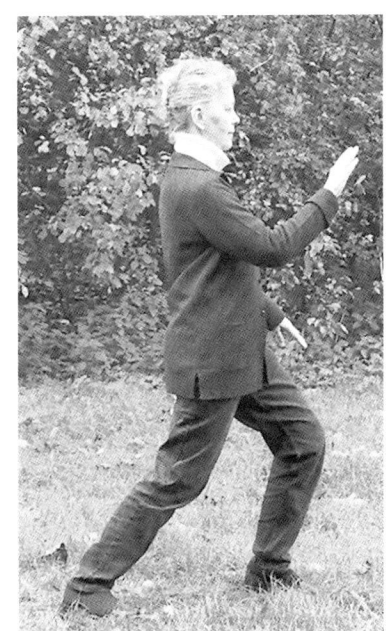

PLAYING THE GUITAR

Shift all your weight into the left foot. Right foot comes off the ground, step back on to it, ball down first. Transfer weight into right foot as right hand comes down, left comes up into Playing the Guitar, right palm facing left elbow. With left toes off the ground, the left heel comes into line with the right heel as you bring the arms closer to each other.

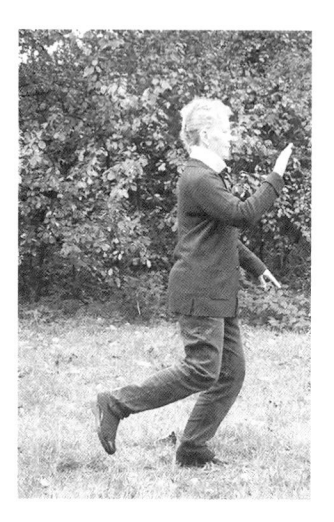

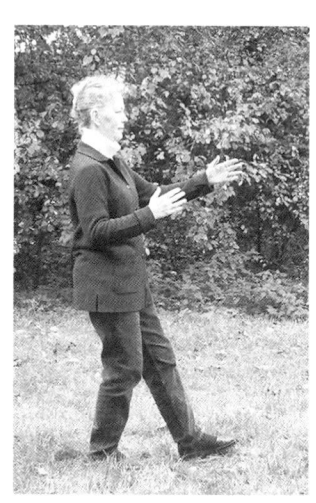

BRUSH LEFT KNEE AND TWIST STEP

Turn to the right, turning on the heel of the left foot as the right hand comes down, round, back and up to ear height. Simultaneously the left hand goes across, round and down. Step out onto the left foot, brush knee with left hand, strike with right. 70% weight in front foot, back foot 45° angle. You are now facing west.

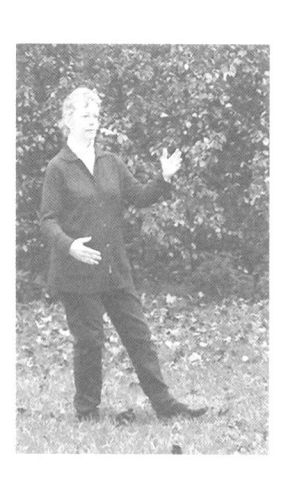

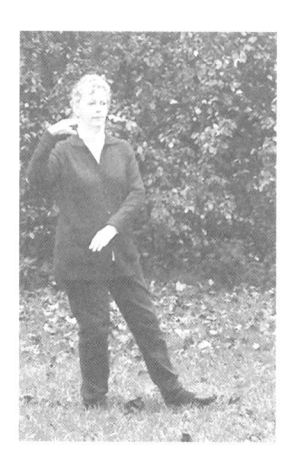

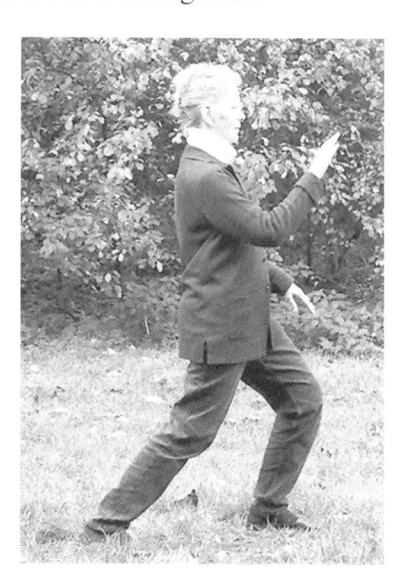

STEP FORWARD, DEFLECT DOWNWARD, INTERCEPT AND PUNCH

Shift weight back into the right foot, turn to the left lifting the ball of the left foot. Right hand comes down below navel, palm facing up, the left arm is by your left side, also with palm facing up. The right hand is higher than the left. Step onto left foot, make fist with the right hand. Step to the northwest corner with the right foot, hands come round in front of you, left palm in front, right fist by your right hip. Left foot comes forward, shoulder width. Body facing northwest. As you shift the weight into the left foot the right fist comes forward in an arc, then a straight line as you strike with the fist, while the left hand comes down and back to behind right wrist. 70% weight in the left foot.

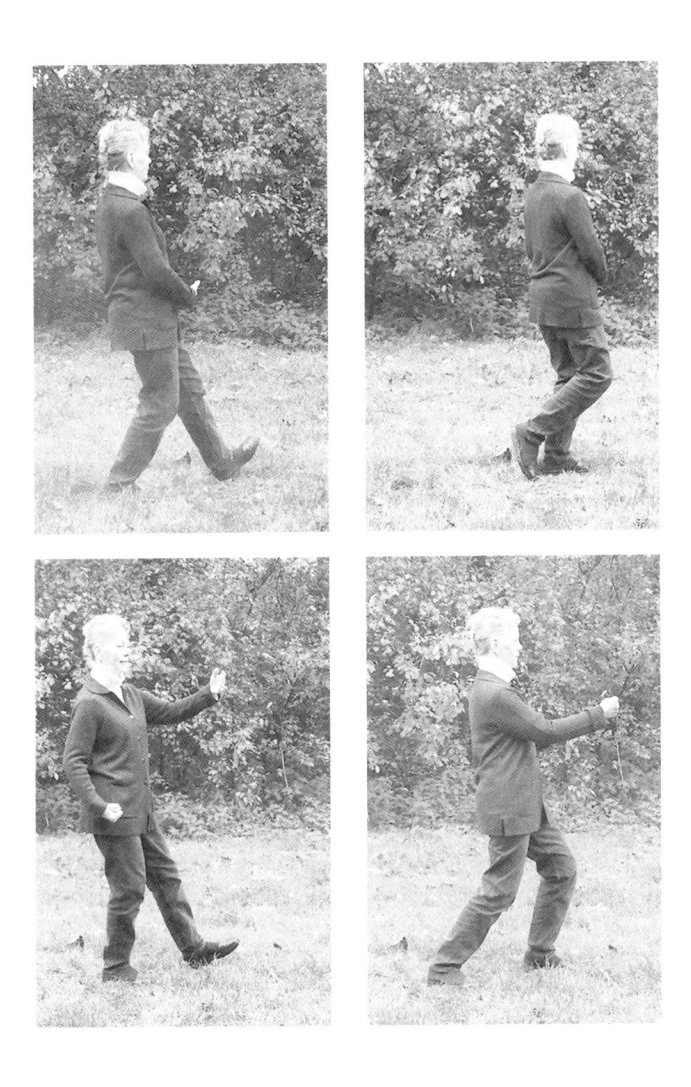

WITHDRAW AND PUSH

Keeping the weight distribution the same turn the hips to the left, the right hand opens as the arm extends. Turn the hips back as you sit onto the right foot as the right hand passes through the left elbow joint. All the weight is now in your right leg. Shift weight forward into left foot, push with the hands, chest height and chest width, until 70% of your weight is in the front leg.

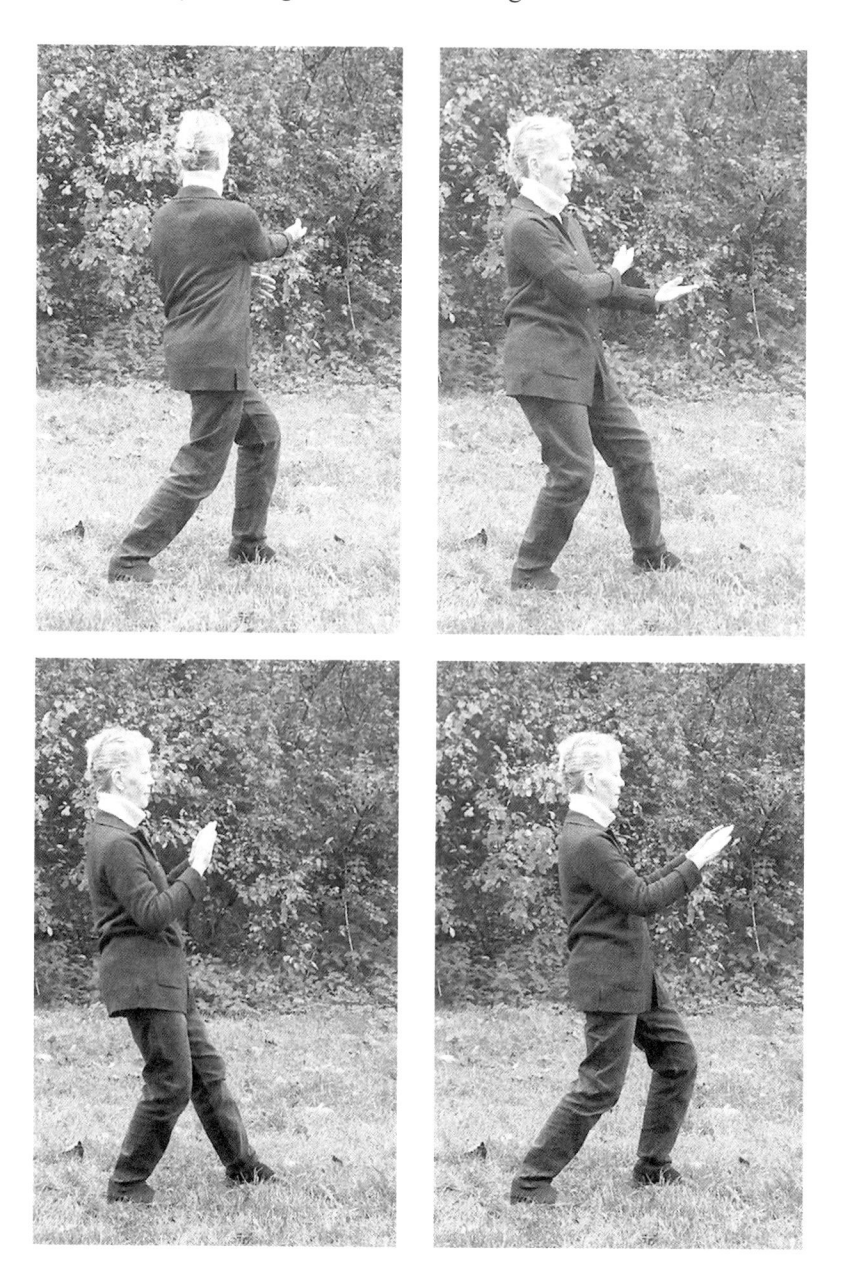

Side view from the Punch

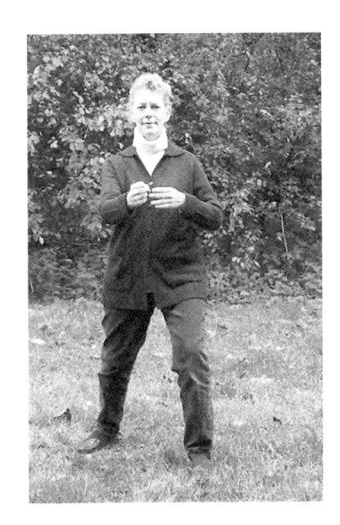

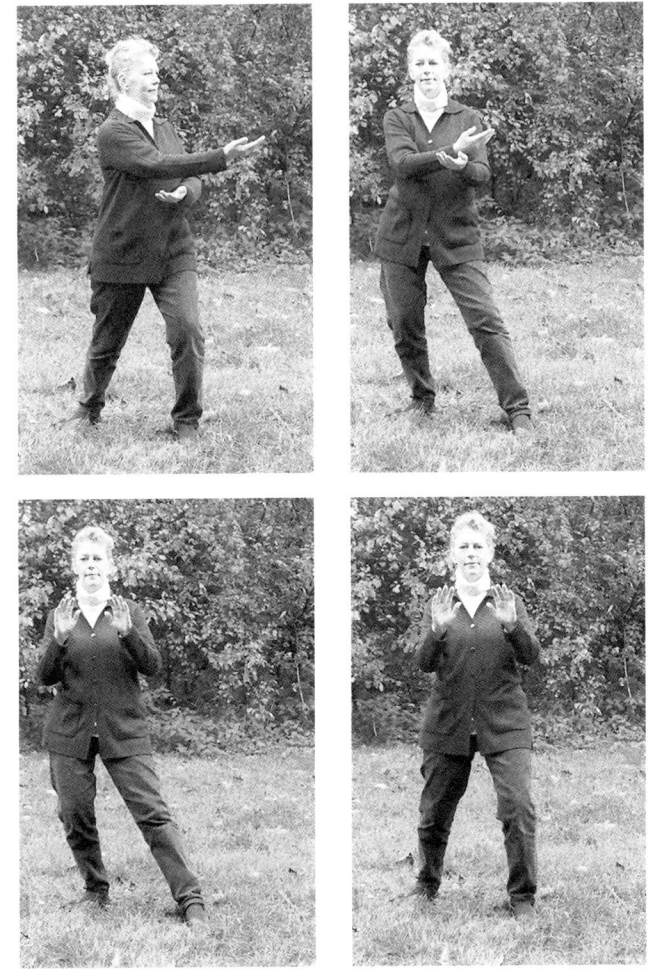

CROSSING HANDS

Sit back onto your right leg as you turn to the right, right hand circles out as you turn your left toes 90°. Shift all the weight onto the left foot as you turn on the ball of the right, the left hand goes out and down in a circle, right foot steps back in line with left as the arms come round in a circle and meet at the wrists, chest height, right in front of left, palms facing body, crossing at wrists. 80% of weight in left foot and 20% in right.

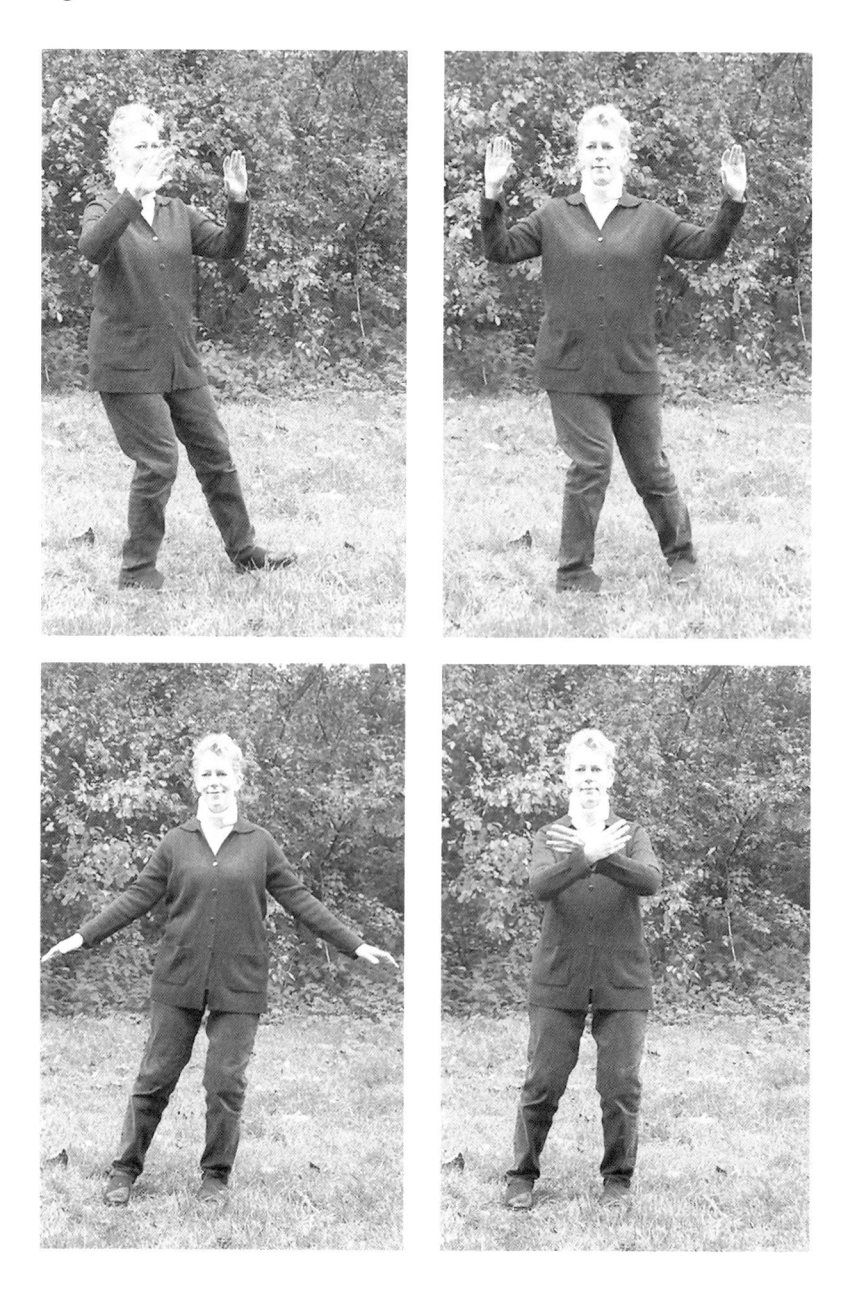

Side view of Crossing Hands

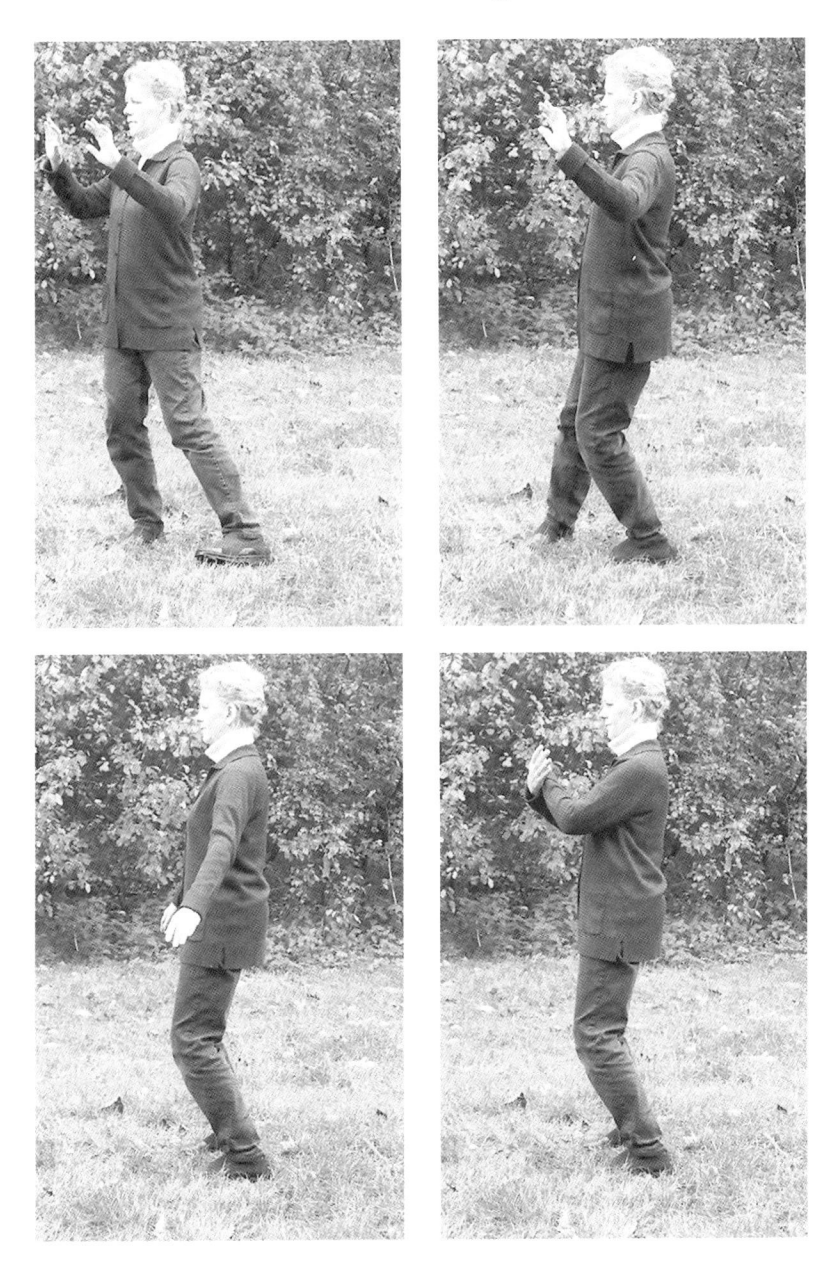

EMBRACE THE TIGER TO RETURN TO THE MOUNTAIN

Sink all your weight into your left foot as you turn on the ball of your right foot, both hands come down still in contact at the back of the wrists, right palm facing down, left facing up. The left hand circles down round and up to left ear as you begin to step behind you to the southeast corner with the right foot, heel first. Shift weight into the right foot as you brush knee with the right hand, strike with the left, as the back toes turn in 45°. At the last moment the right palm turns up. 70% weight in right foot.

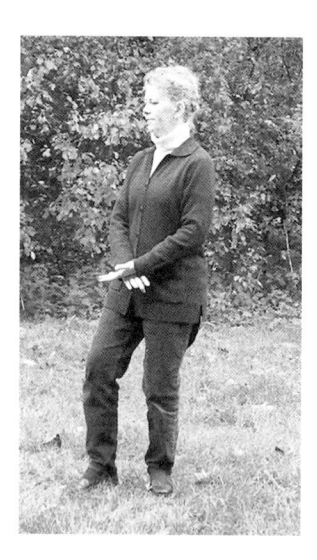

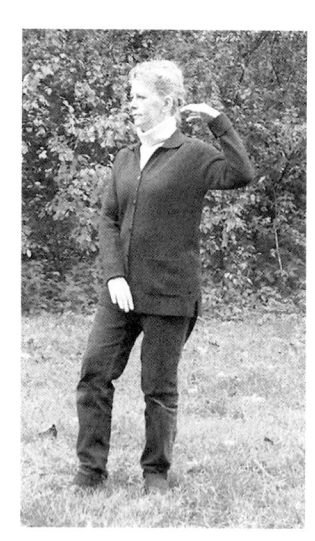

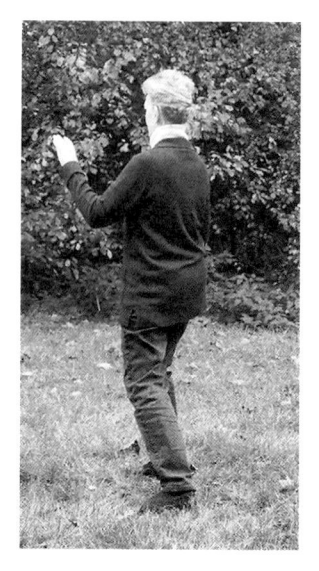

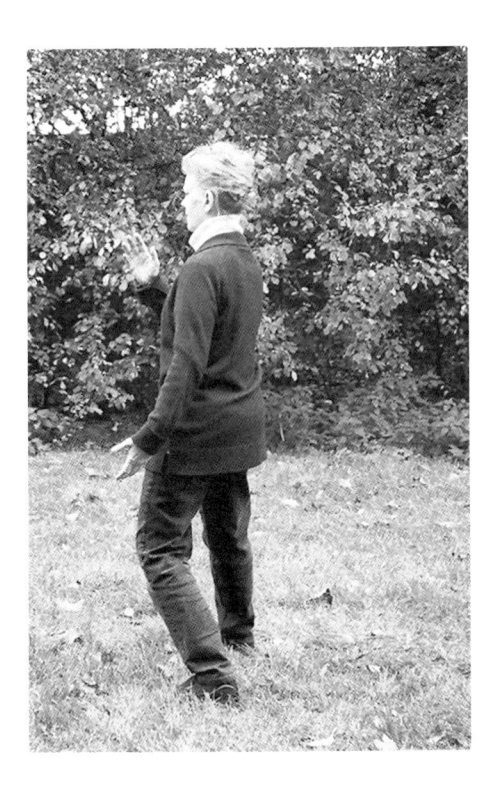

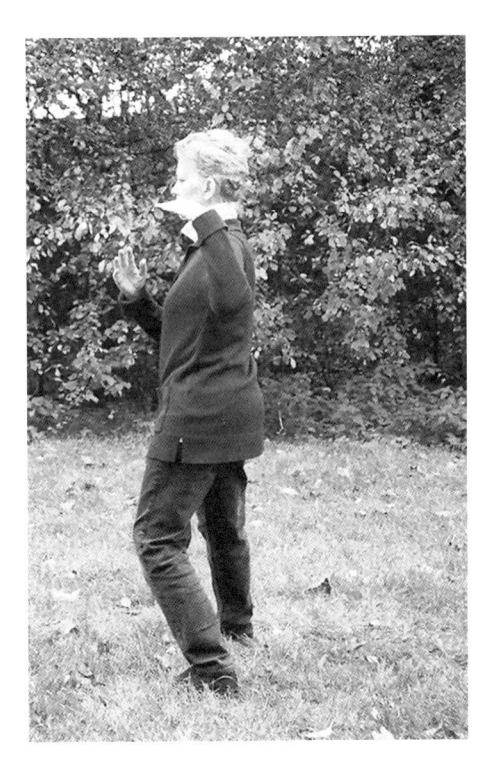

GRASP THE SPARROWS TAIL ROLL BACK

Sit back onto your left leg. As you turn, the left hand comes down round and up in an arc of a circle to ear height, while the right hand comes in front of your body. All your weight is in your left foot.

GRASP THE SPARROW'S TAIL PRESS

Shift weight back into the right foot as the left palm comes forward to touch the right inner wrist, chest height, hips straight. 70% of weight in right foot.

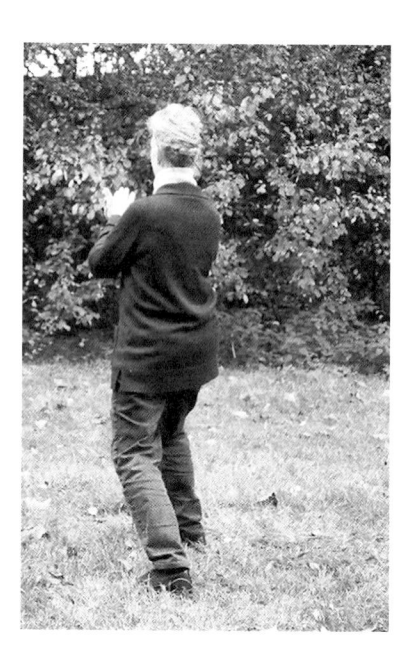

GRASP THE SPARROW'S TAIL PUSH

Sit back onto the left leg, hands separate, shift into your right leg, push with the hands, fingertips shoulder height and chest width, elbows bent. 70% of your weight on the front leg.

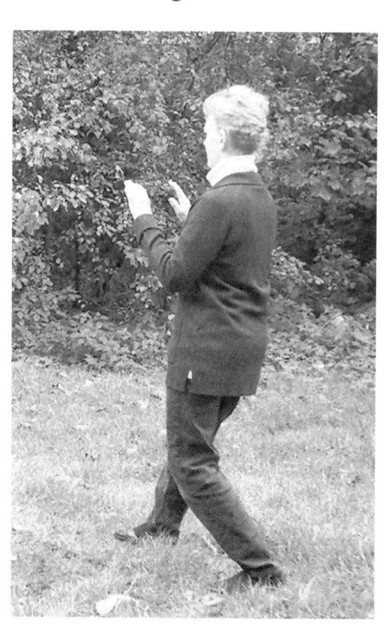

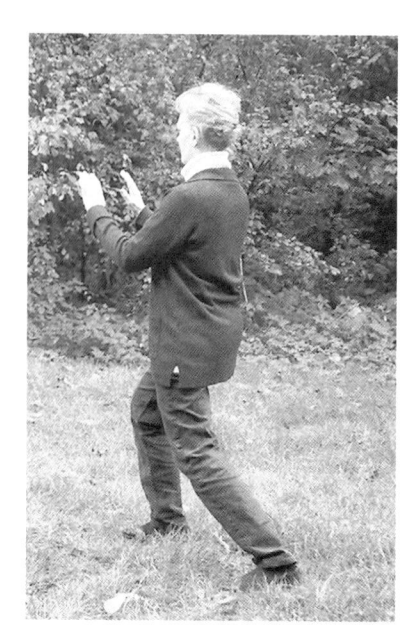

SINGLE WHIP FACING THE CORNER

Sit back onto your left leg, the arms come down parallel to the ground, elbows slightly bent, all the weight is in your left leg. Turn your torso and the right toes to the left as far as they will go, your nose, navel and arms maintaining the same relationship to each other. Shift the weight back into the right foot as you turn the waist to the right. Left hand comes down with the palm facing up underneath the right hand, all the fingers of which are joined in the shape of a bird's beak, all the weight on your right foot. Turn the hips to the left and pivot on the ball of the left foot, the right hand moves out to the east, shoulder height. Step out widely to the northwest corner onto your left heel. Shift the weight into the left foot, the left hand rises in front of you, turn your waist to the northwest, the right toes turn in at an angle of 45°, at the last moment the left palm turns over.

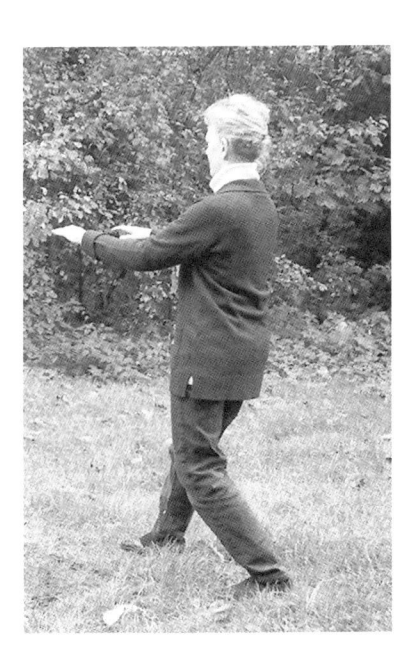

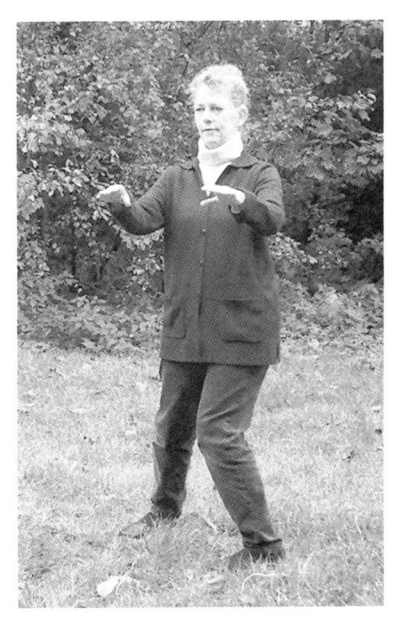

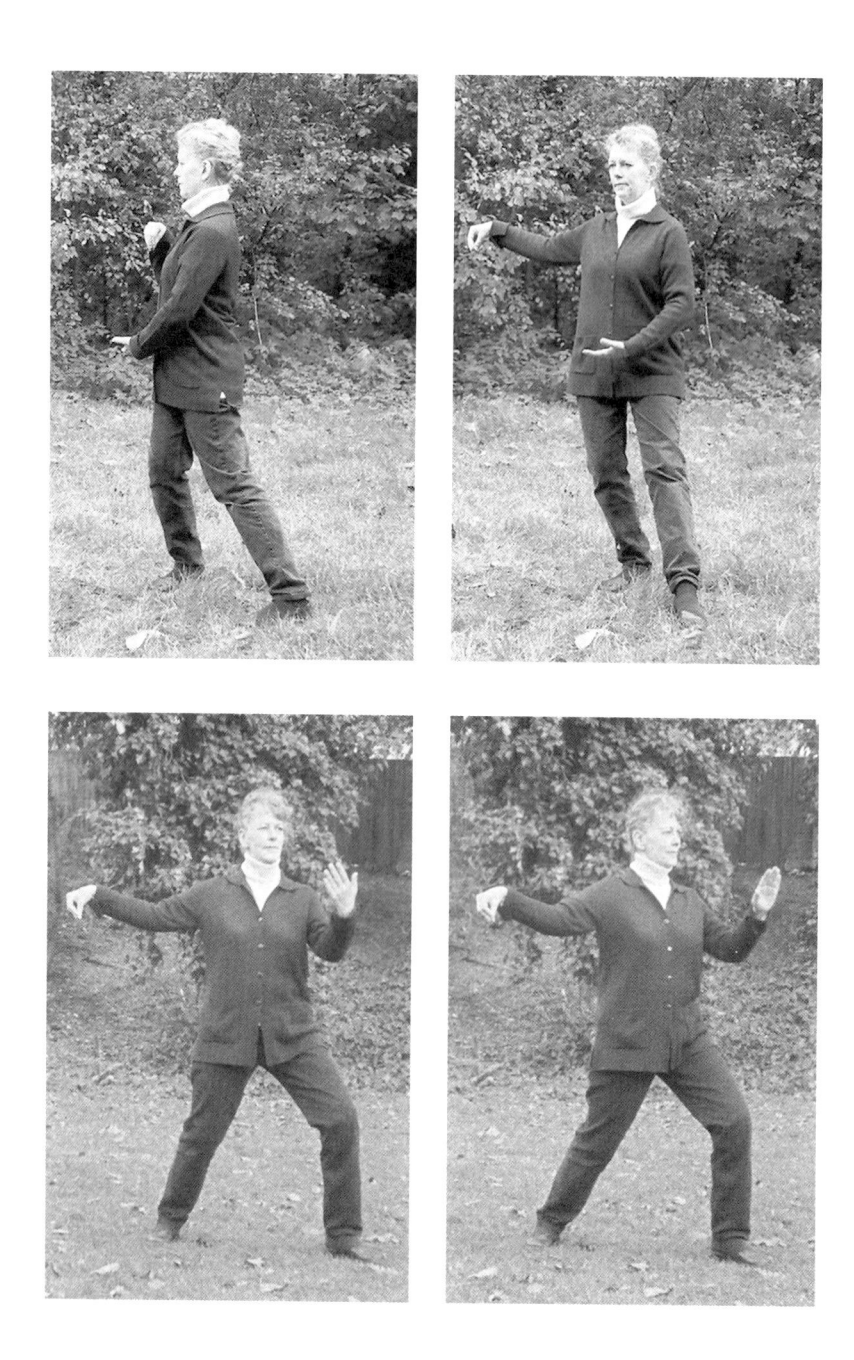

FIST UNDER ELBOW

Sit back onto the right leg, the beak opens, turn torso to the west, step out onto the left heel, the inside of the arms face each other, shift the weight onto your left leg, turn hips to right and turn on the ball of the right foot, arms remain in the same relationship, move right heel in line with left heel, turn torso to northwest, place foot down at angle of 45° to the corner, shift weight into right, turn hips to left, turn on the ball of the left foot. As you turn the hips to the right, left hand moves round slightly behind you and comes up as the left foot advances forward to rest on the heel, toes pointing up. The right hand comes down to form a fist underneath left elbow.

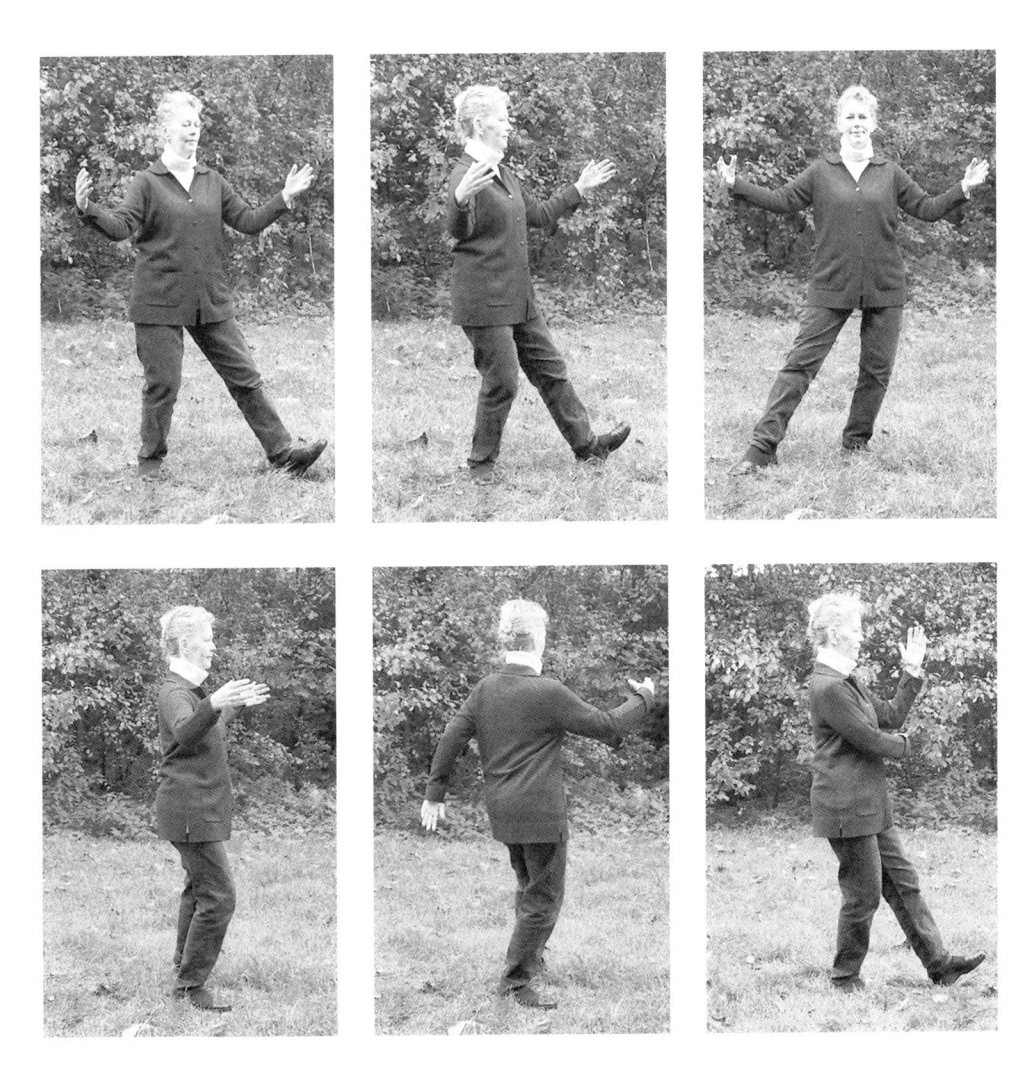

REPULSE MONKEY

Turn to the right. Fist opens, right hand moves round in an arc of a circle while the left hand goes forward.

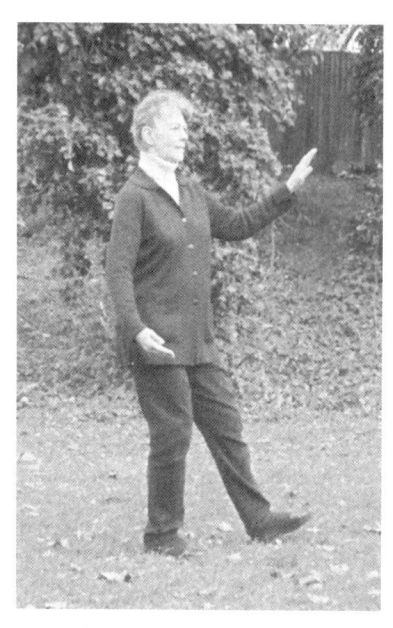

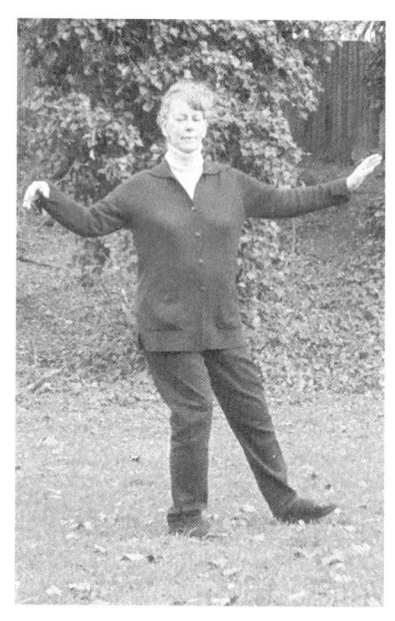

As you turn the hips to the left, both palms turn over, right palm faces down, ear height, while left palm faces up. Step back onto the ball of a parallel left foot, shoulder width. Shift the weight into the left foot, as you do so the left hand comes down by your thigh, the right hand moves forward and the right toes turn straight, waist straight.

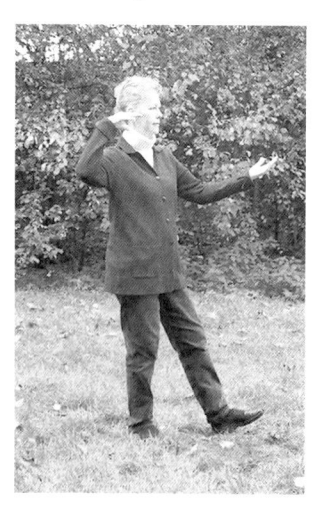

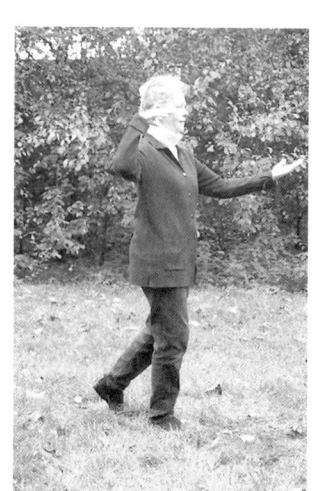

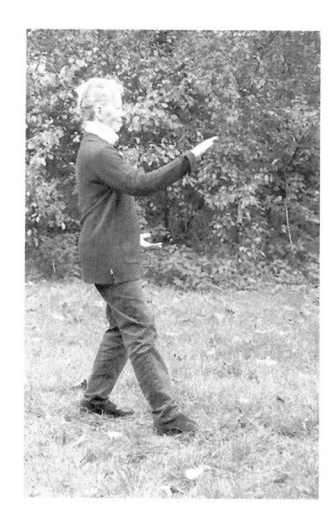

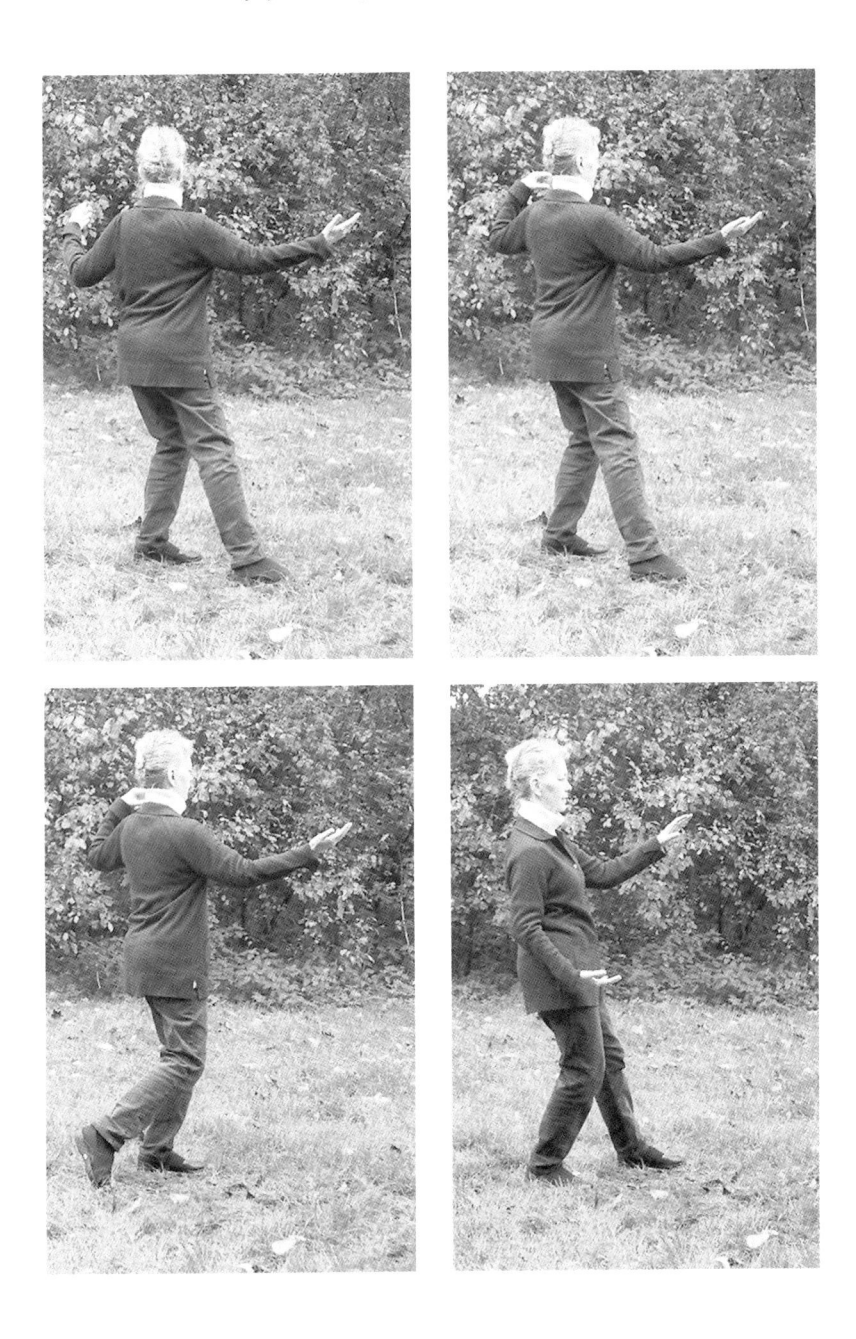

Turn to the left, left hand moves round in an arc of a circle, while the right hand goes forward. As you turn the hips back to the right, both palms turn over, left palm faces down, ear height, while right palm faces up. Step back onto the ball of the parallel right foot, shoulder width, shift weight into right foot, as you do this, the right hand comes down by your thigh, the left hand moves forward, waist straight.

Turn to the right. Right hand moves round in an arc of a circle while the left hand goes forward. As you turn the hips to the left both palms turn over, right palm faces down, ear height, while left palm faces up. Step back onto the ball of the parallel left foot, shoulder width. Shift the weight into the left foot, as you do so the left hand comes down by your thigh, the right hand moves forward, waist straight.

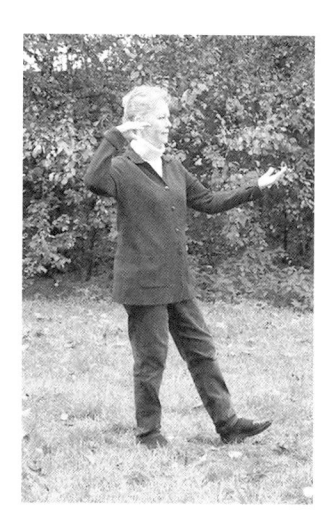

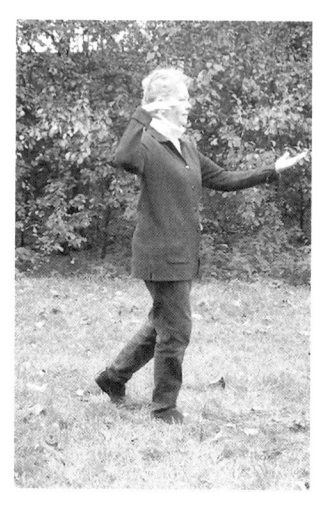

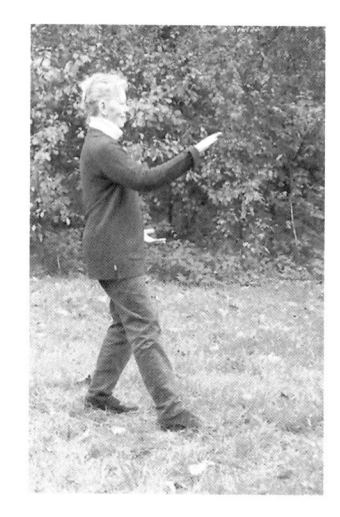

Turn to the left, left hand moves round in an arc of a circle, while the right hand goes forward. As you turn the hips back to the right, both palms turn over, left palm faces down, ear height, while right palm faces up. Step back onto the ball of the parallel right foot, shoulder width, shift weight into right foot, as you do this, the right hand comes down by your thigh, the left hand moves forward, waist straight.

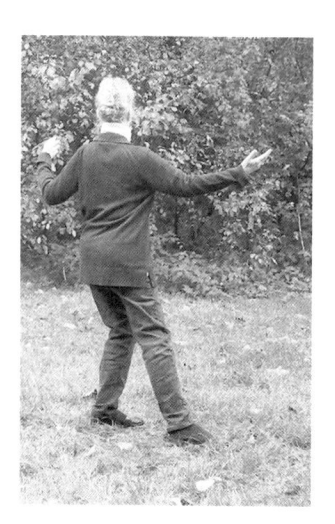

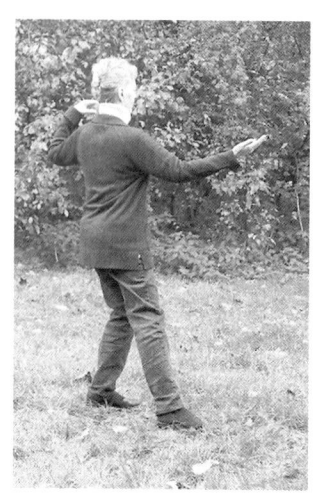

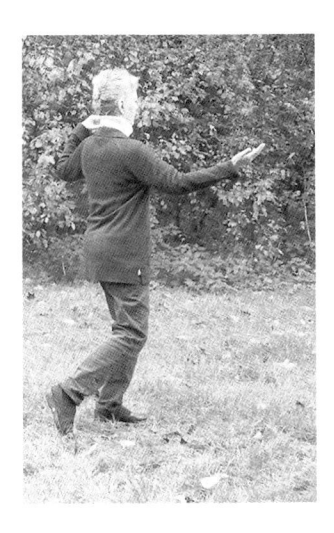

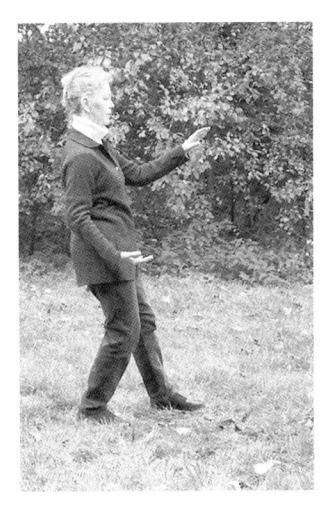

Turn to the right. Right hand moves round in an arc of a circle while the left hand goes forward. As you turn the hips to the left, both palms turn over, right palm faces down ear height, while left palm faces up. Step back onto the ball of the parallel left foot, shoulder width. Shift the weight into the left foot, as you do so the left hand comes down by your thigh, the right hand moves forward, waist straight.

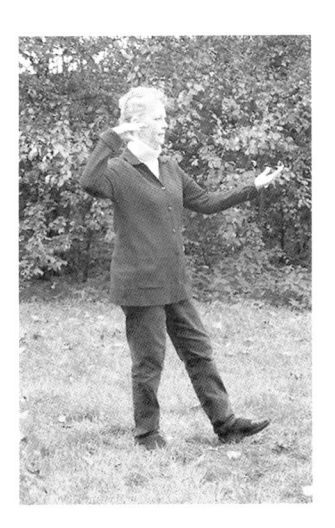

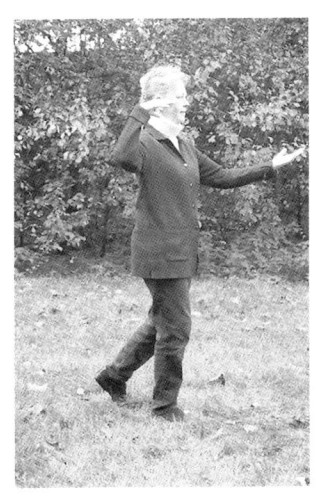

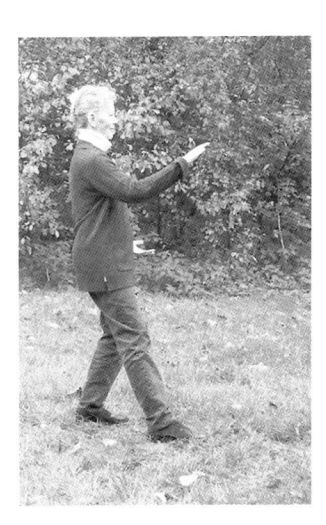

DIAGONAL FLYING

All the weight on the left foot, turn to the left, left hand goes up, right hand comes down in an arc of a circle underneath the left palm.

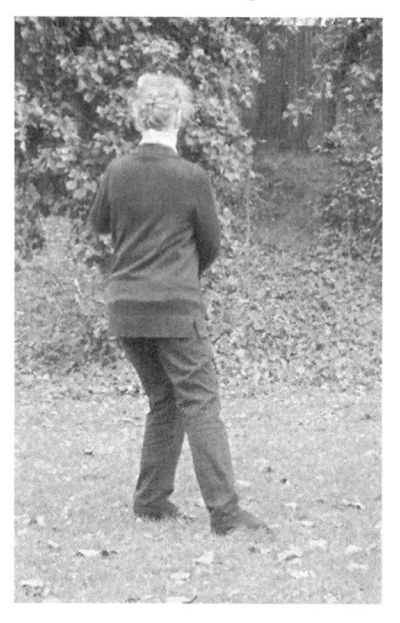

Turn the hips back. Step out behind you onto the right heel to the northeast corner. As you shift into the right foot, the right hand rises face height, palm facing up, the left comes down by your left side, palm facing back, left toes turn in 45°. 70% weight in right leg. Body facing northeast.

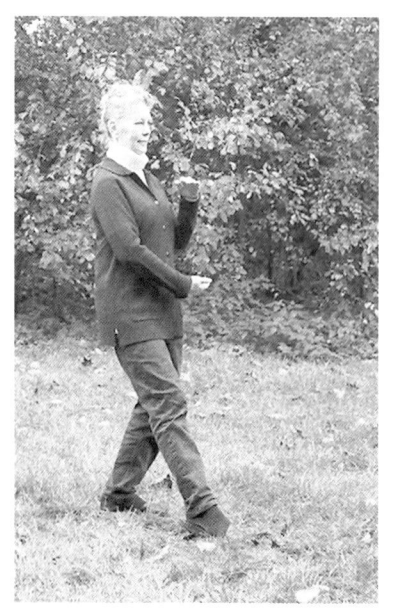

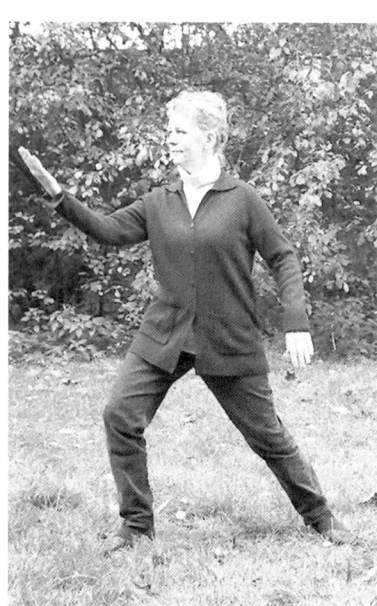

WAVE HANDS IN THE CLOUDS

Shift all your weight into the right foot, turn torso to the east, left palm under the right as left foot comes up parallel to the right, toes straight. All the weight in the right foot. Shift weight into left foot, as you do so the hands change position, the left hand goes on top, the right goes to the bottom, palm facing down. Turn your waist, palms face body, the right foot turns straight, parallel with left.

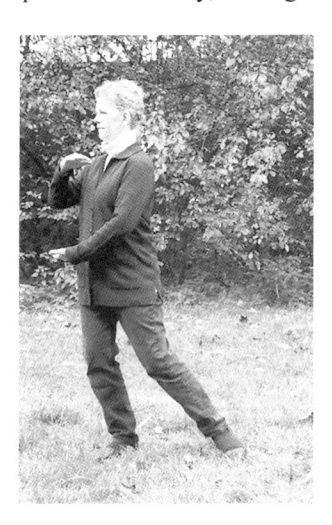

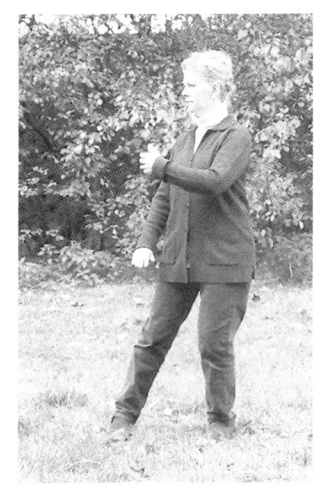

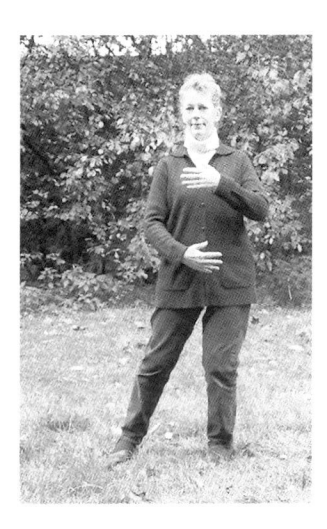

Continue to turn the waist, the palms face each other, all the weight is in the left leg. Bring the right foot next to the left, less than shoulder width. Shift the weight into the right foot, as you do so the hands change position as the right hand goes on top the left hand goes to the bottom, palm facing down.

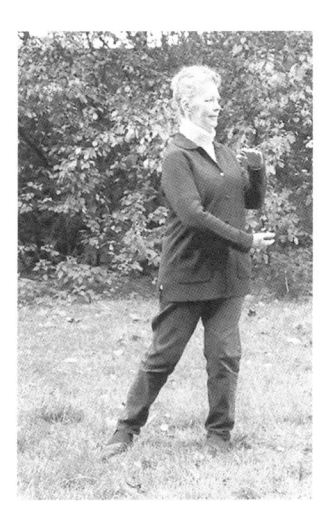

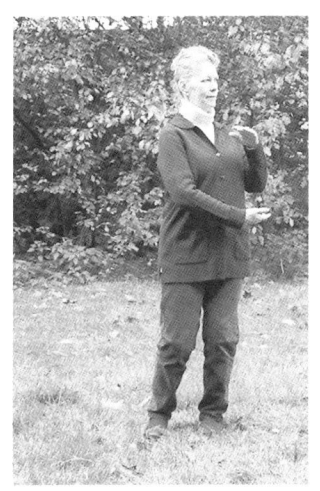

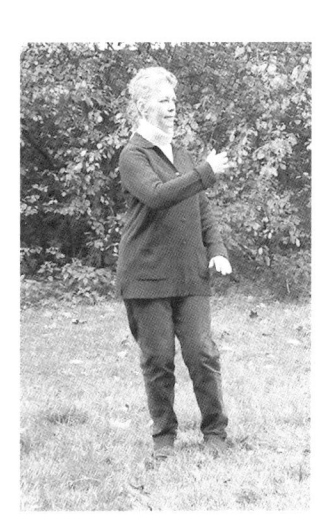

Turn your waist, the palms face you, continue to turn the waist, palms face each other, right on top, left on bottom. All the weight in the right leg. Lift left foot away from right, wider than shoulder width.

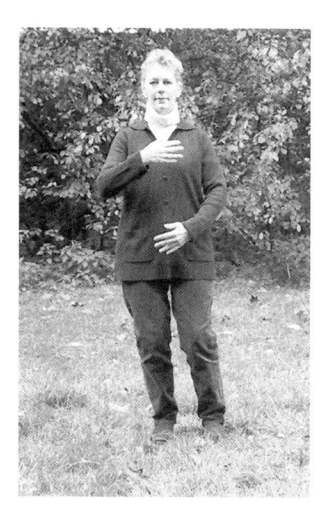

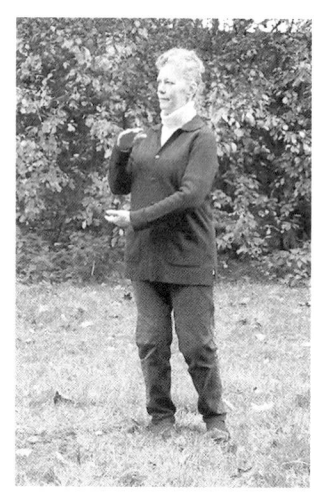

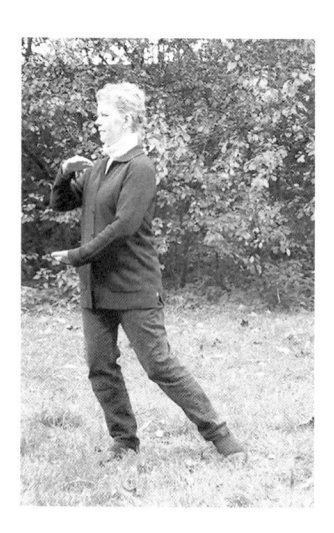

Move weight into left foot, as you do so the hands change position, as the left hand goes on top, the right goes to the bottom, palm facing down. Turn waist palms face you, continue to turn waist, the palms face each other, all the weight is in the left leg.

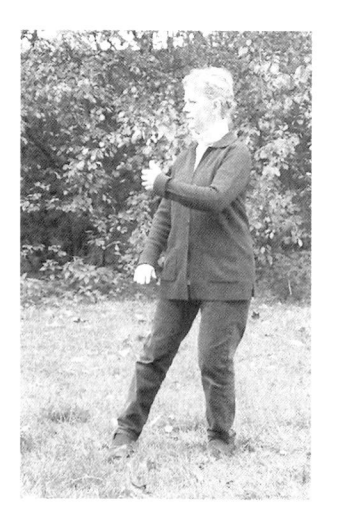

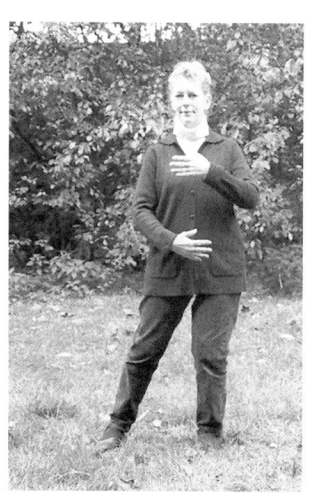

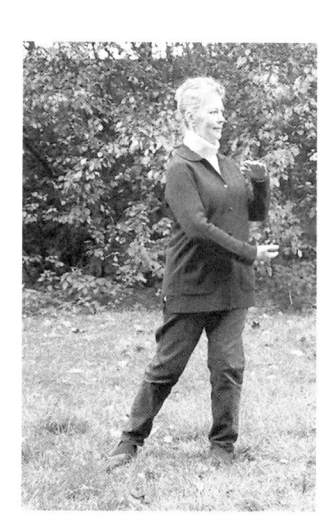

Bring the right foot next to the left, less than shoulder width. Shift the weight into the right foot, as you do so the hands change position as the right hand goes on top the left hand goes to the bottom, palm facing down. Turn your waist, the palms face you.

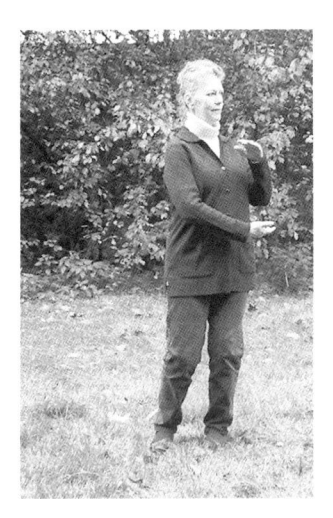

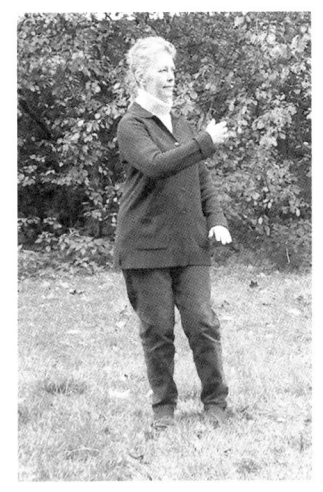

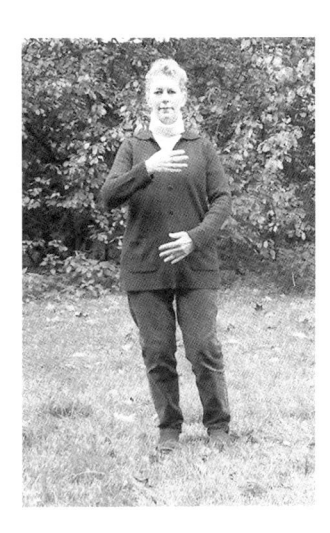

Continue to turn the waist, palms face each other, right on top, left on bottom. All the weight in the right leg. Lift left foot away from right, wider than shoulder width. Move weight into left foot, as you do so the hands change position, as the left hand goes on top, the right goes to the bottom, palm facing down.

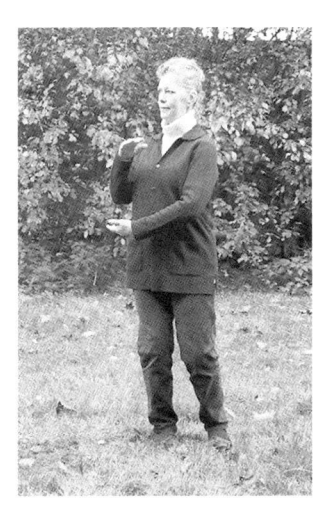

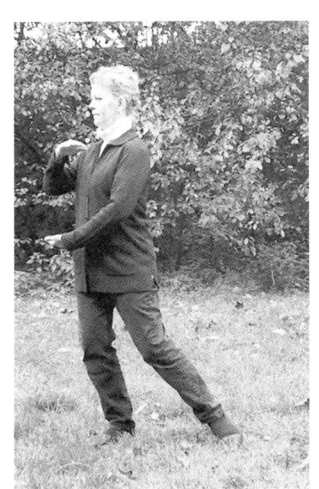

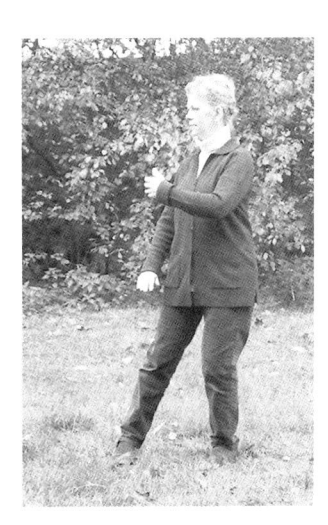

Turn waist, palms face you, continue to turn waist, the palms face each other, all the weight is in the left leg, body facing northwest.

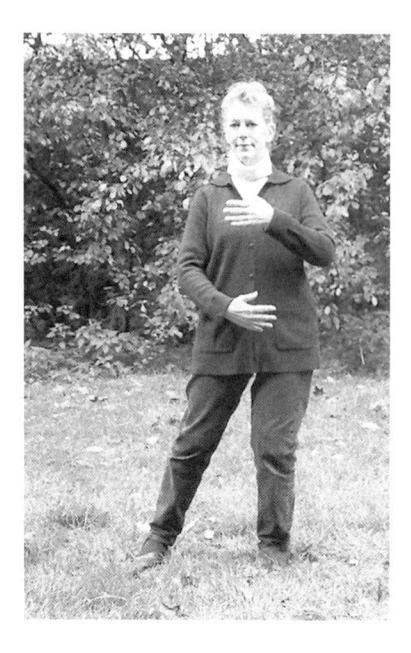

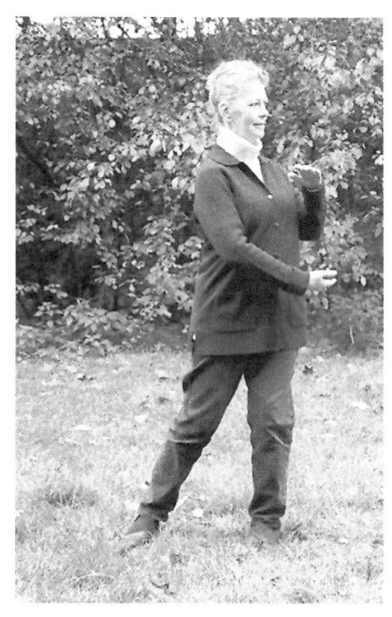

SINGLE WHIP

Step out onto the right heel and as you shift weight into the right foot, right hand comes up, wrist bent to shoulder height as the fingers come together to form a beak. Left hand comes down to below the navel, palm facing up, left foot turns on the ball.

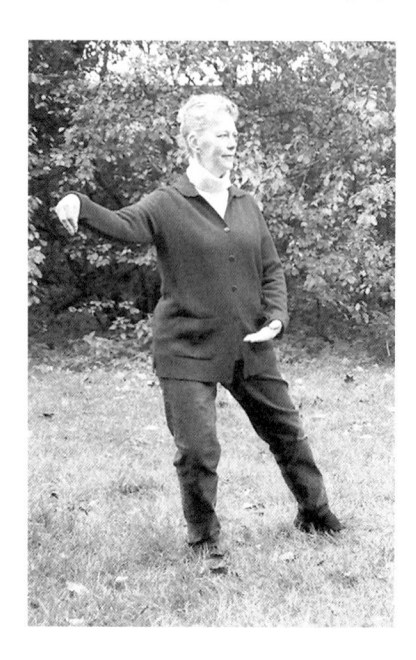

Step out widely onto your left heel, shift into the left foot, the left hand rises in front of you, turn your waist to the west, the right toes turn in at an angle of 45°, at the last moment the left palm turns over. 70% weight in left foot, shoulder width between heels.

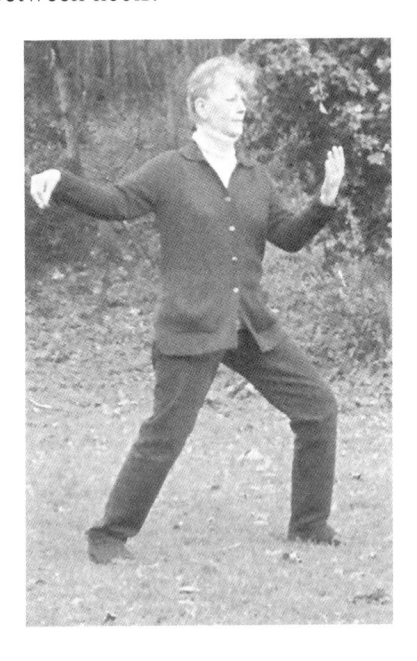

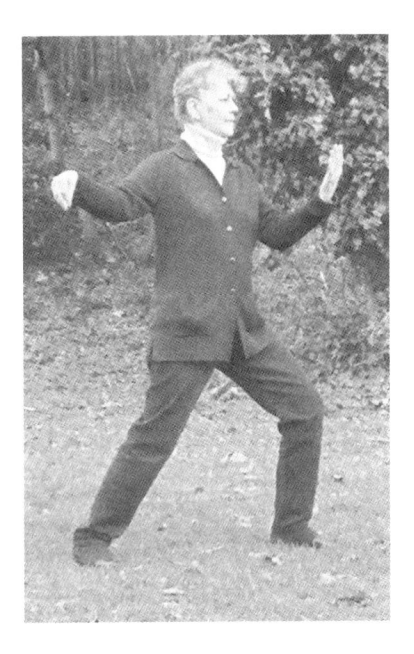

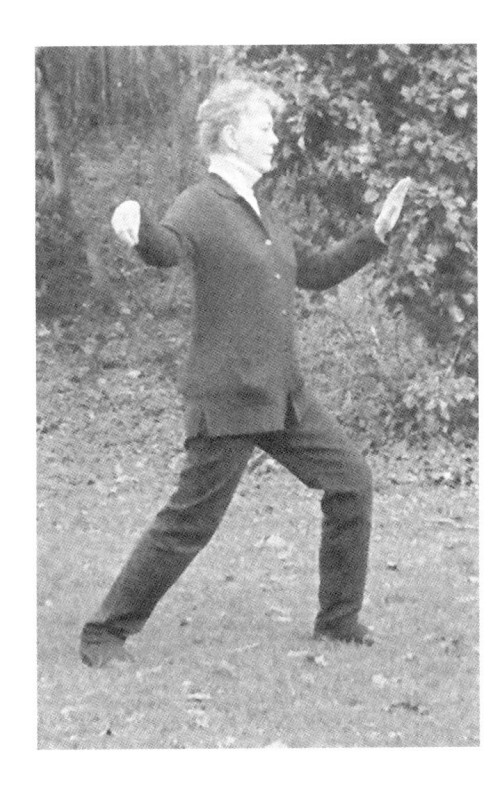

SNAKE CREEPS DOWN - SQUAT SINGLE WHIP

Turn to the right, as the right toes and left palm turn to the right. Sit back and sink for the Snake Creeps Down. The left hand comes back slightly, fingers pointing forward, turn the left toes in 45°. As you shift the weight into the left foot the left hand moves forward on the inside of the left thigh. Left toes turn out 90° to the corner.

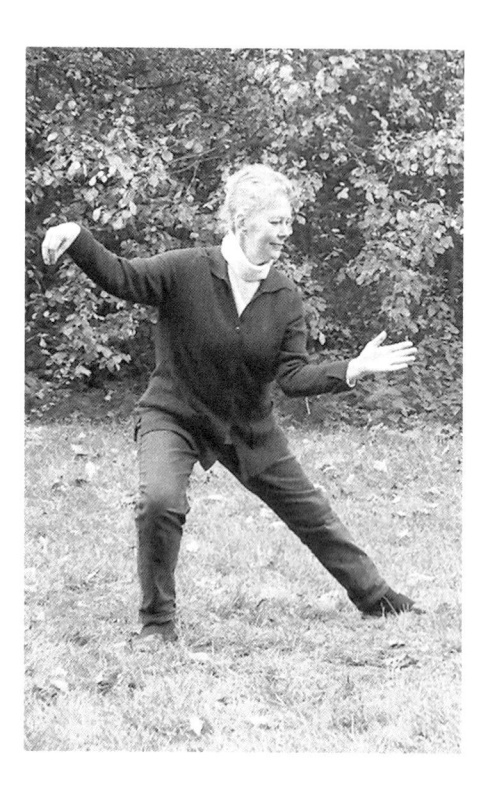

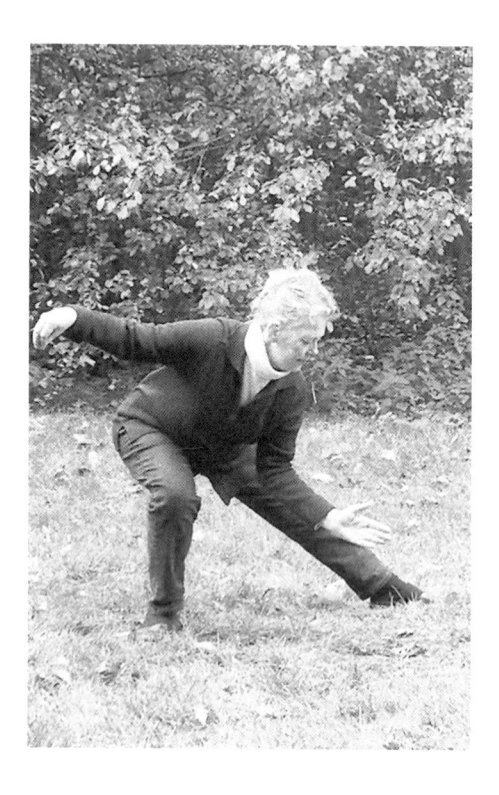

GOLDEN COCKEREL STANDS ON LEFT LEG

When around 70% weight is in left foot, right toes have come in 45°. Left hand moves up to face height as beak comes down to behind right thigh. Come up 100% onto left leg, left hand comes down to left thigh as right hand opens and comes up simultaneously with the right leg. Knee navel height, toes pointing down.

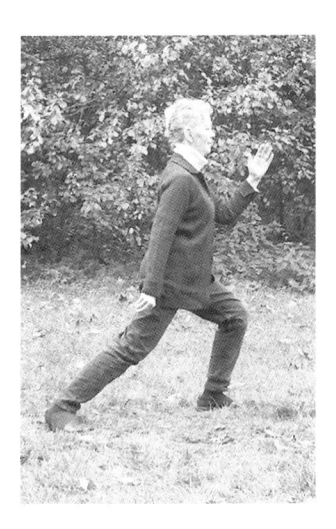

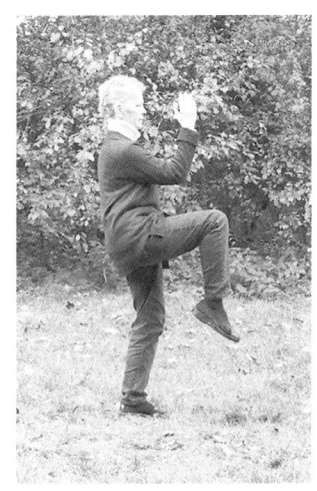

GOLDEN COCKEREL STANDS ON RIGHT LEG

Step back onto right leg, ball first, right hand comes down to right thigh as left comes up, finally the left knee lifts to navel height with the toes pointing down.

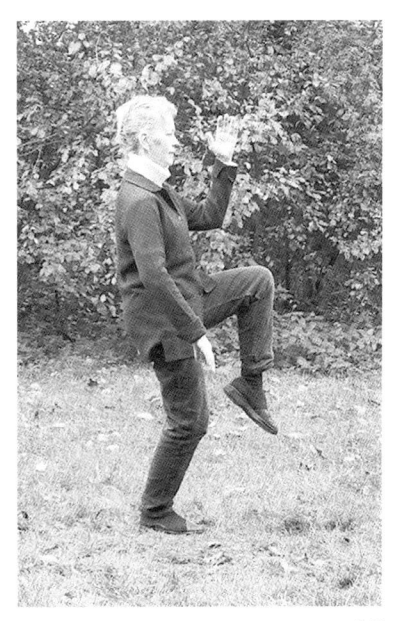

SEPARATE THE RIGHT FOOT

Step back onto the ball of the left foot. As the weight goes into the left foot, right hand comes up around and forward throat height palm facing down, while the left hand comes down, palm facing up resting in front of left thigh. All the weight is now on the left leg, right foot is resting on the ball (this is not a posture but a stage between two postures). Turn your waist to the left, the hands come down and round in circles, turn waist to the right, the arms complete their circles meeting at the wrists, chest height, left resting on top of right, both palms facing body. Reverse the position of the palms, hand separate, kick with right toes to knee height, bottom of foot parallel with floor, right hand chopping northwest, left to south, eyes looking northwest. This is the first of the low kicks.

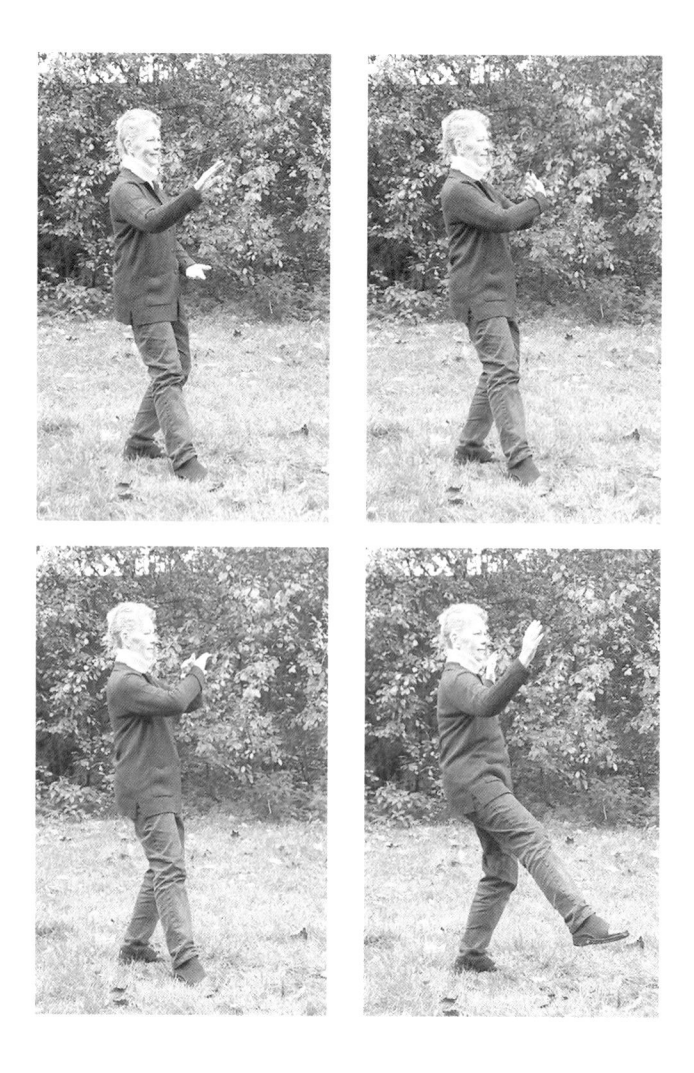

SEPARATE THE LEFT FOOT

Step to the northwest corner onto right foot, weight moves into right as right hand comes down in front of right thigh, palm up, left hand comes down slightly and turns to face southwest, throat height, palm facing down, eyes face southwest (this is not a posture but a stage between two postures). As you transfer 100% of weight to right foot turn waist to the right, hands come down and round in circles, left foot moves from behind to front, resting on ball, pointing southwest, turn waist to left, the arms complete their circles meeting at the wrists, chest height, right resting on top of left, palms facing body, reverse the position of the palms. Hands separate, kick with left toes to knee height, bottom of foot parallel with floor, left hand chopping southwest and right to north, eyes looking southwest. This is the second of the low kicks.

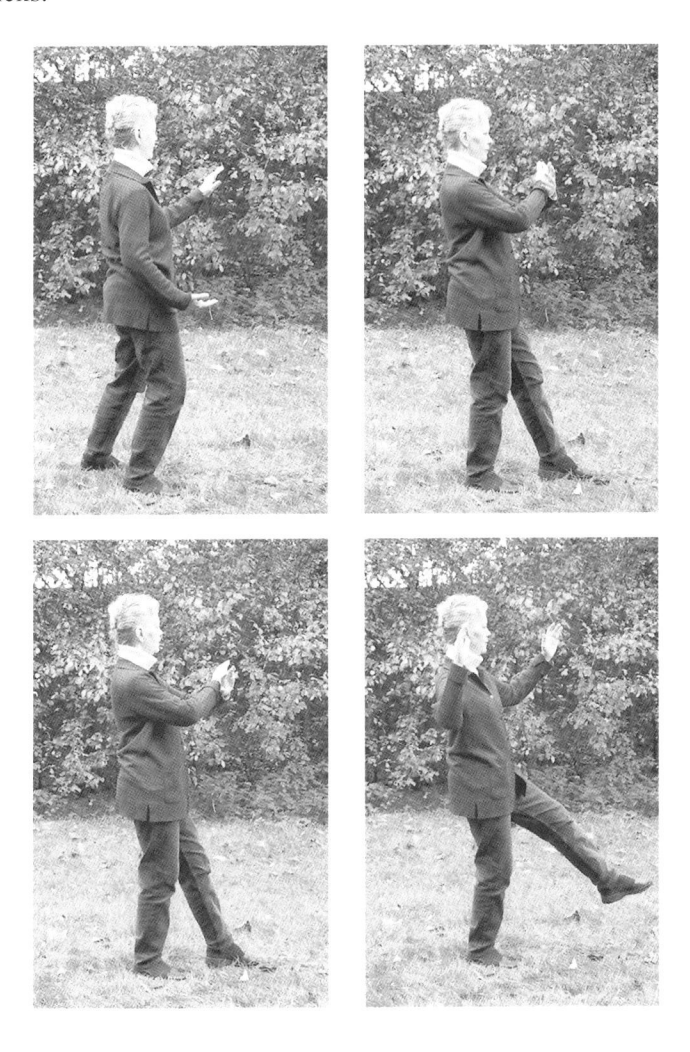

TURN AROUND AND STRIKE WITH HEEL

As left toes relax down, turn torso to northwest, then using your right arm to propel, swing to the left on the heel of the right foot 180° so that the right toes point to southeast. Arms come together at wrists, neck height, right resting on top of left, both palms facing body. As left foot and left knee rise, palms face away from body, left toes come up, high kick with the left heel straight forward as the left hand chops down to east and the right to southwest.

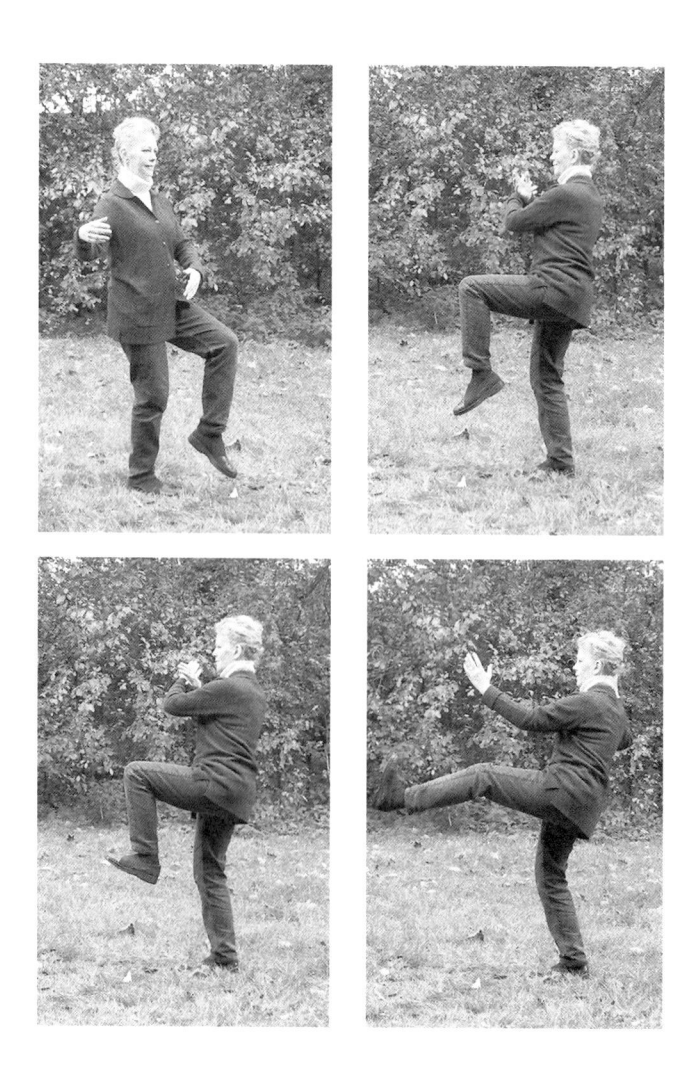

BRUSH LEFT KNEE

Bring foot back, step out to east, shoulder width between heels. The left hand comes down to right hip while right hand comes to ear height, step, brush knee with left hand, strike with the right.

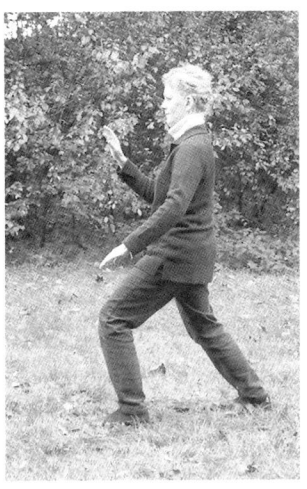

BRUSH RIGHT KNEE

Sit back onto the right foot as the body turns to northeast, left toes come up and turn out 45° to the left, right hand comes to left shoulder, palm facing down, while left palm faces up by left thigh. As you shift weight into left foot, right hand comes down to left thigh and the left hand comes up to ear height. Step forward onto the right foot to the east, feet shoulder width apart. Brush knee with right hand, strike with left.

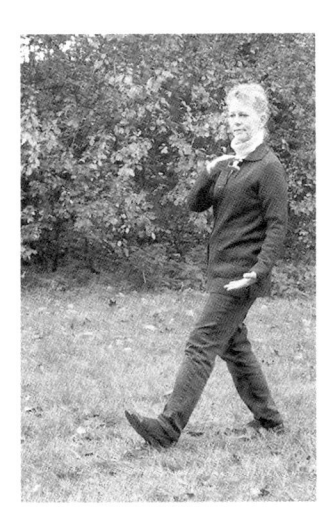

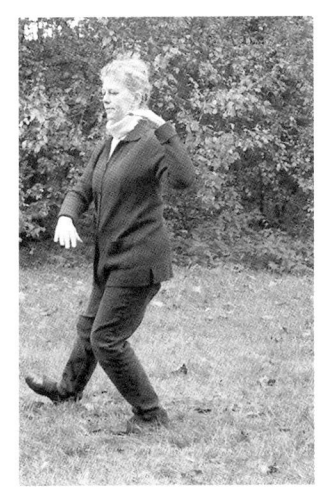

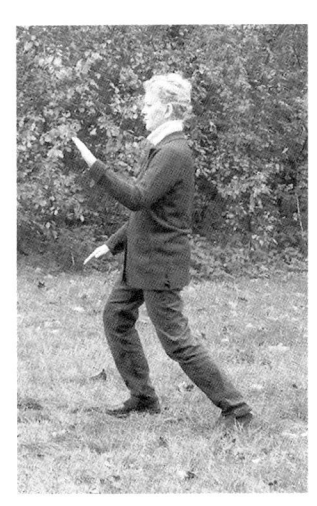

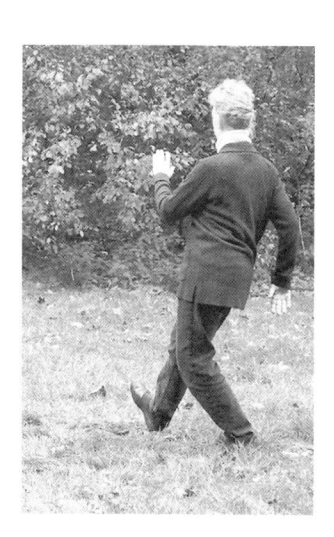

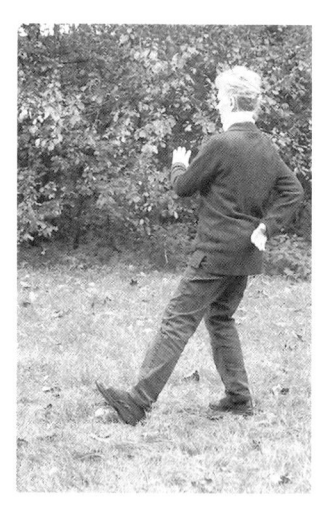

STEP FORWARD AND STRIKE WITH FIST

Sit back onto the left foot, as you turn to the right, right toes come up and turn out 45° to the right. Shift weight into right foot. Step to the east with left foot shoulder width, form fist with right hand, shift weight into the left foot, brush knee with left hand, low punch with right, body inclines forward with a straight back, 70% weight in front leg.

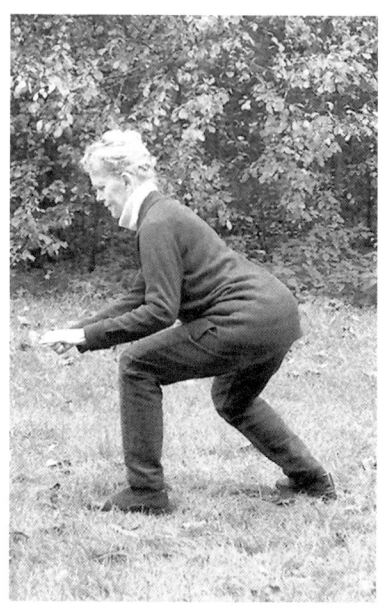

STEP FORWARD AND WARD OFF RIGHT

Sit back on the right leg, body upright, right hand opens as left hand comes closer to right hand, left toes turn out 45°. Step forward onto the left leg, then step onto the right, shoulder width, weight shifts into right foot as hands come up to chest height. Left fingers pointing at right palm in ward off, 70% of weight in front foot.

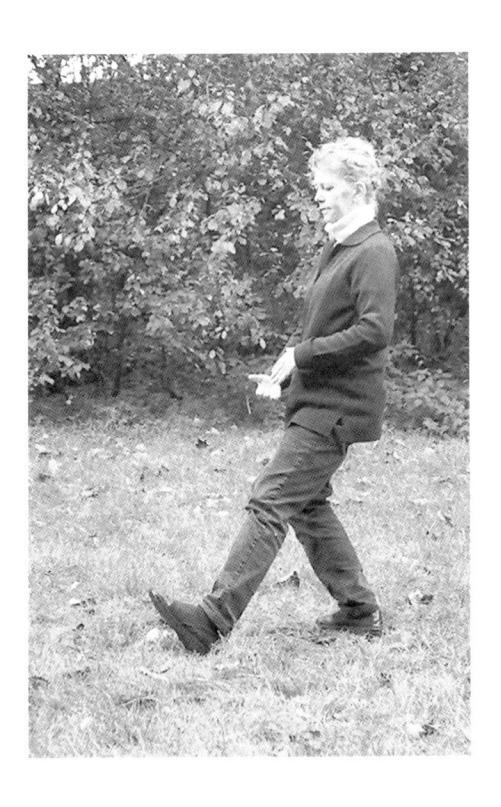

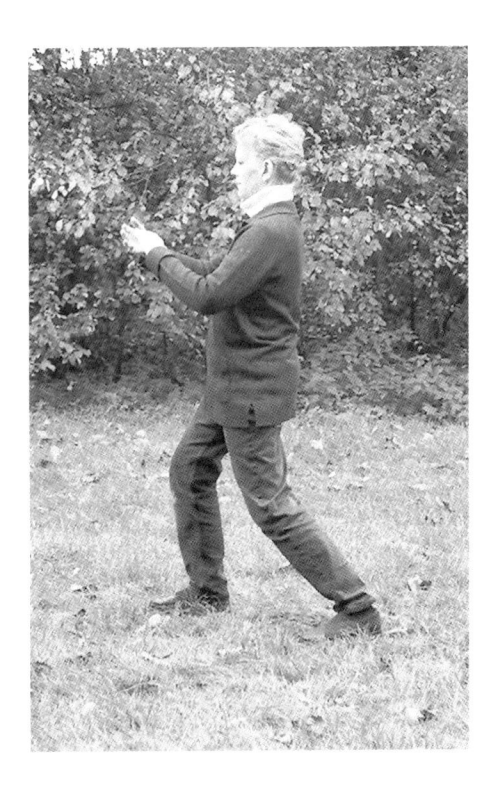

GRASP THE SPARROW'S TAIL ROLL BACK

Turn your waist to the right 10°, keeping the weight distribution the same. Sit back onto your left leg. As you turn, the left hand comes down round and up in an arc of a circle to ear height, while the right hand comes in front of your body. All your weight is in your left foot.

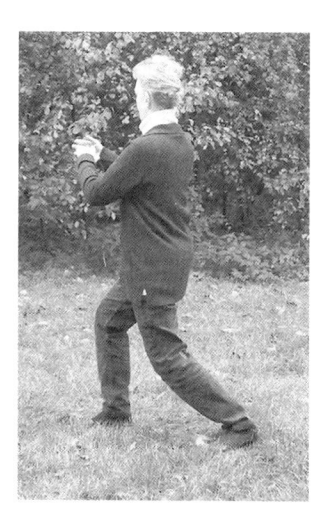

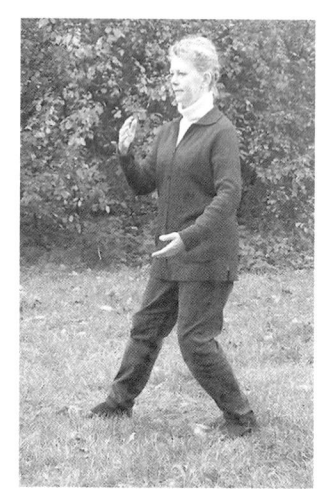

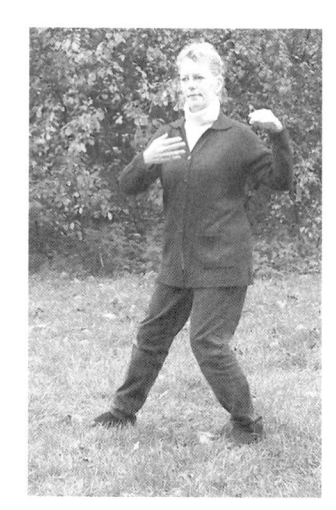

GRASP THE SPARROW'S TAIL PRESS

Shift weight back into the right foot as the left palm comes forward to touch the right inner wrist, chest height, hips straight. 70% of weight in right foot.

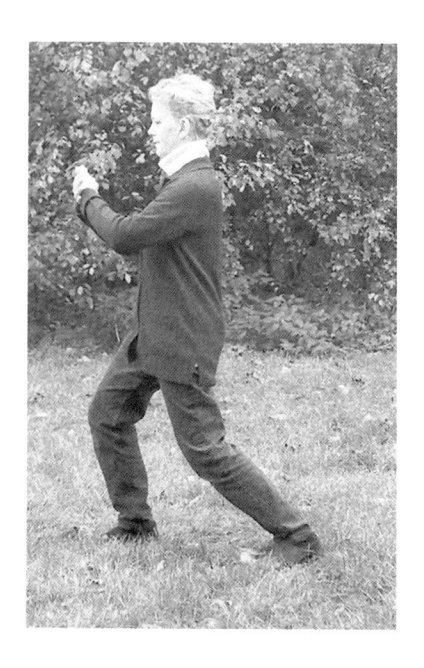

GRASP THE SPARROW'S TAIL PUSH

Sit back onto the left leg, hands separate, shift into your right leg, push with the hands, fingertips shoulder height and chest width, elbows bent. 70% of your weight on the front leg.

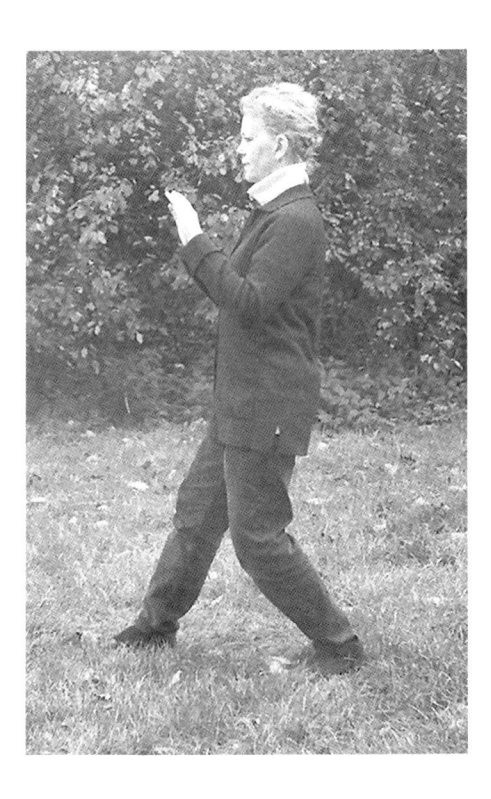

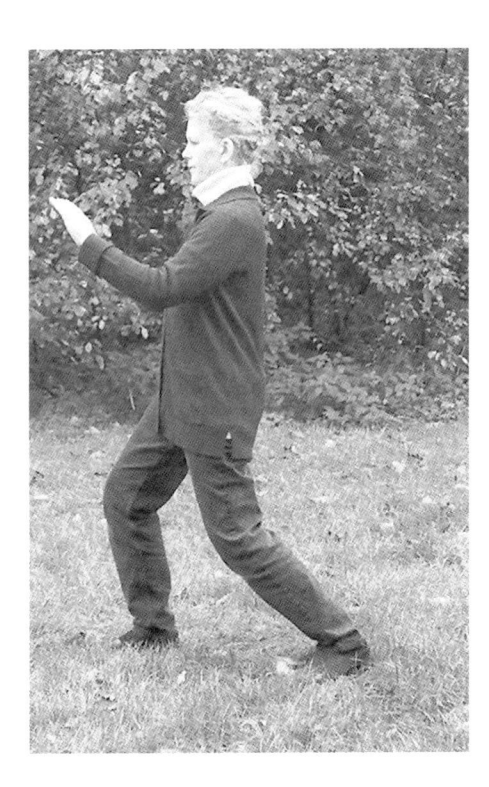

SINGLE WHIP

Sit back onto your left leg, the arms come down parallel to the ground, elbows slightly bent, all the weight is in your left leg. Turn your torso and the right toes to the left as far as they will go, your nose, navel and arms maintaining the same relationship to each other. Shift the weight back into the right foot as you turn the waist to the right. Left hand comes down with the palm facing up underneath the right hand, all the fingers of which are joined in the shape of a bird's beak. All the weight is on your right foot. Turn the hips to the left and pivot on the ball of the left foot, the right hand formed as a beak moves out to the corner, shoulder height. Step out widely onto your left heel. Shift the weight into the left foot, the left hand rises in front of you, turn your waist to the west, the right toes turn in at an angle of 45°, at the last moment the left palm turns over.

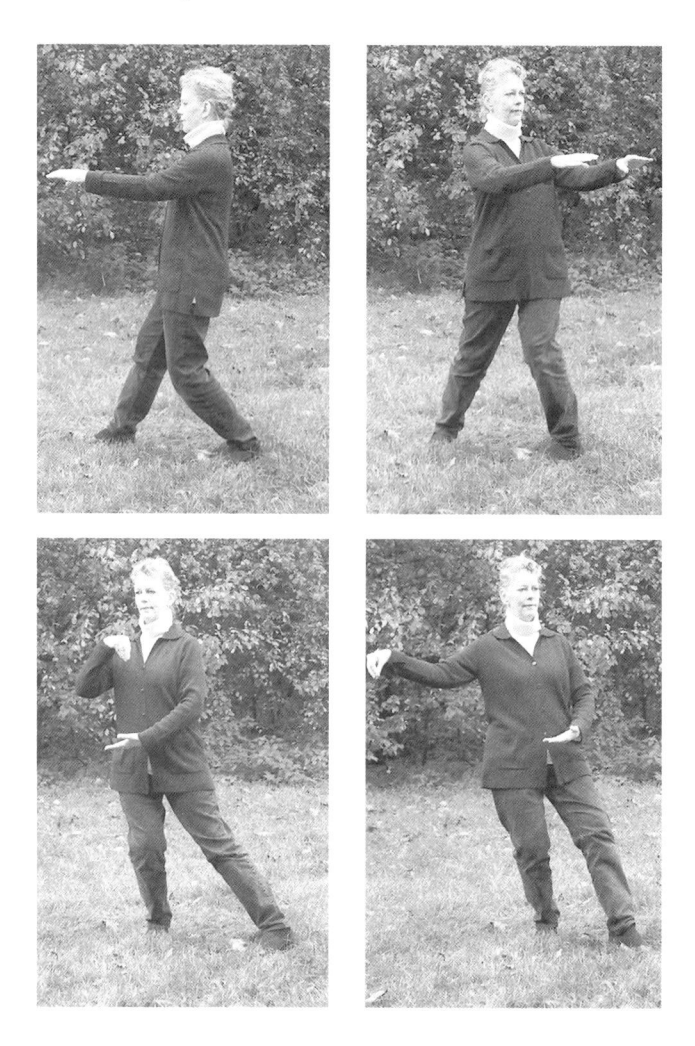

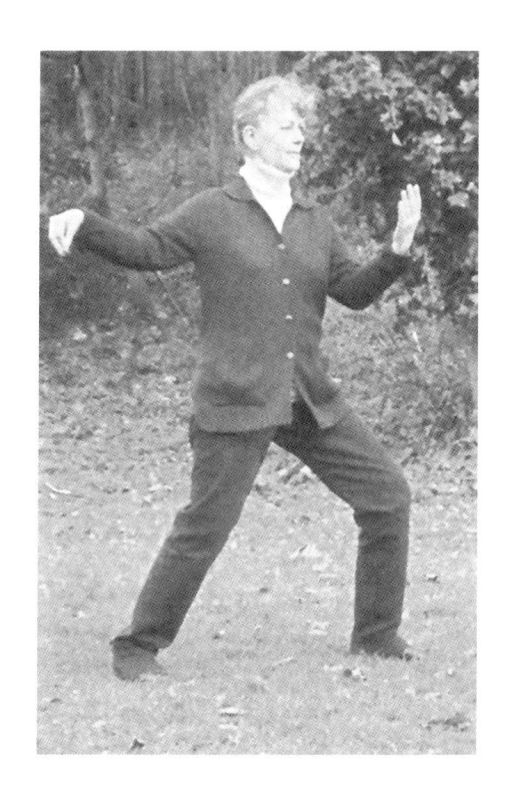

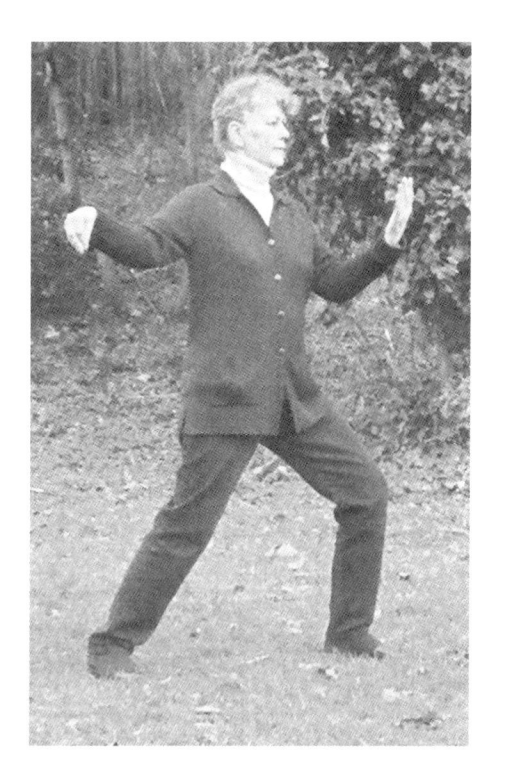

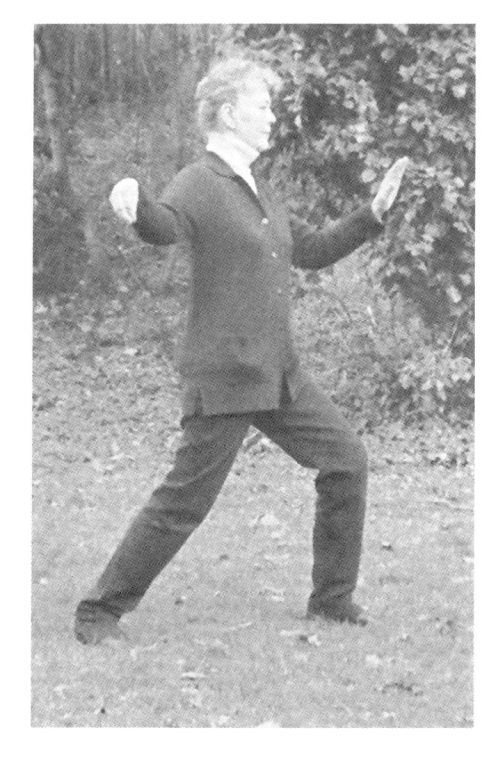

FAIR LADY WEAVING WITH HER SHUTTLE

Shift weight into right foot as you turn the hips to the right, turn the left foot on the heel 90°, at the same time the beak opens and the arms begin to face each other, shift all the weight into the left leg as you pivot on the ball of the right. Simultaneously the right arm bends, fingers open as the left palm comes underneath the right elbow. Step to the east with the right foot, step to northeast with left foot, shoulder width. As the weight shifts into the left foot, the left hand rises up by the left temple, palm turns out, right hand comes forward in a strike, as the hips turn. The right foot turns in 45°. Sit back on the right foot, turn left toes into southeast, pivot on the ball of the right, left arm spirals down, fingers pointing upwards as the right palm comes underneath left elbow, 100% weight in left leg. Step widely behind you onto right heel to northwest, turn the foot, shift weight into the right foot, as right hand rises by the right temple, palm turns out, left hand comes forward in a strike as the hips turn, left foot turns in 45°.

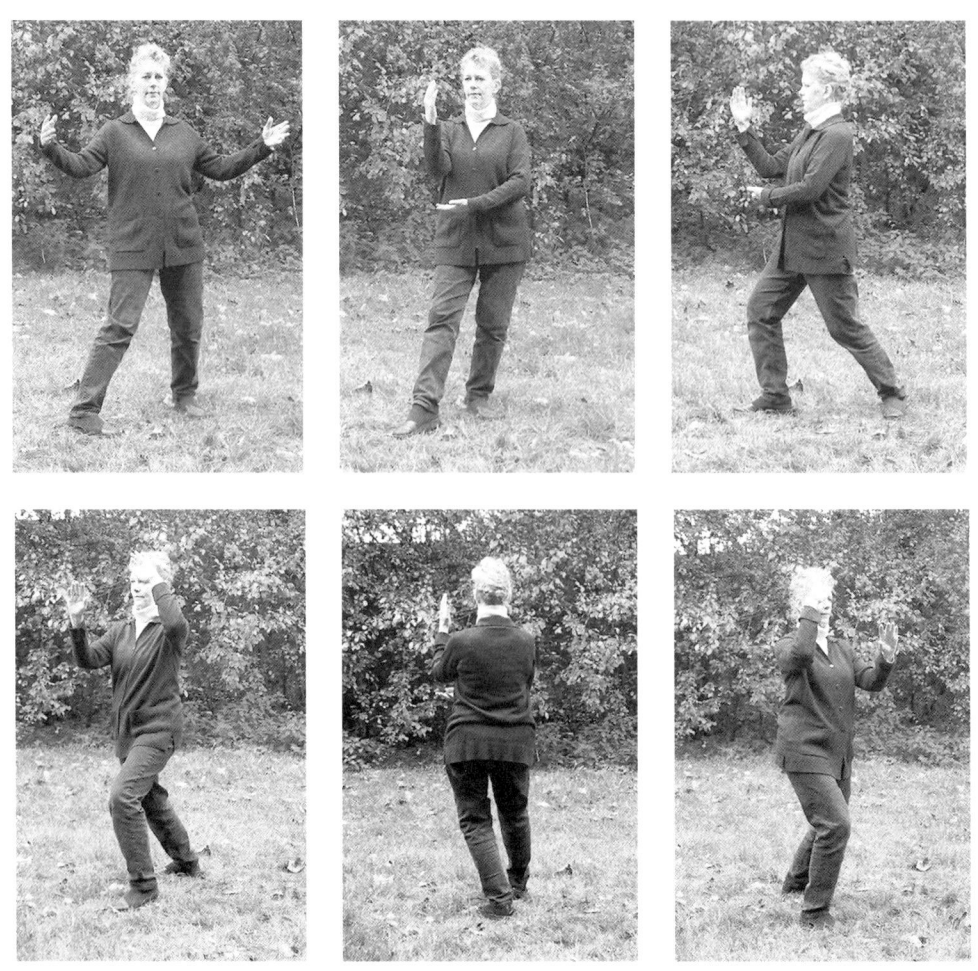

Sit back 100% onto left leg as you rest on ball of right foot, right arm spirals down, fingers pointing upwards as left palm comes underneath right elbow. Step forward to the northwest with right foot, shift weight into right foot, step onto left heel to southwest, shoulder width. Shift weight into left foot, left hand rises by left temple, palm turns out, right hand strikes as hips turn, right foot turns in 45°. Shift weight into right leg, turn left toes to northwest, left arm spirals down, fingers pointing up as right palm comes under left elbow, all the weight goes onto left foot as you turn on the ball of the right foot. Step wide behind you to southeast onto right heel, turn the foot, as weight goes onto right foot, right hand rises by the right temple, palm turns out, left hand strikes, hips turn, left foot turns in 45°.

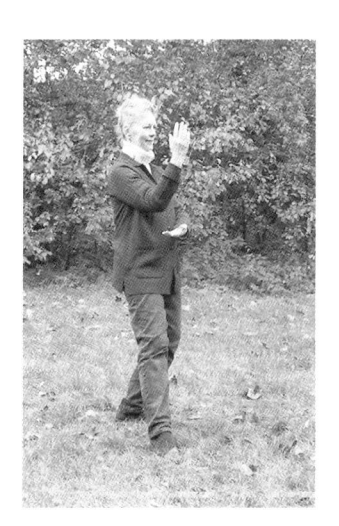

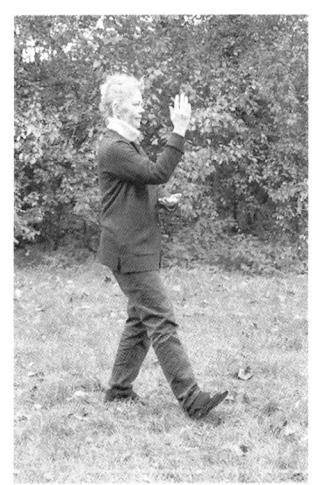

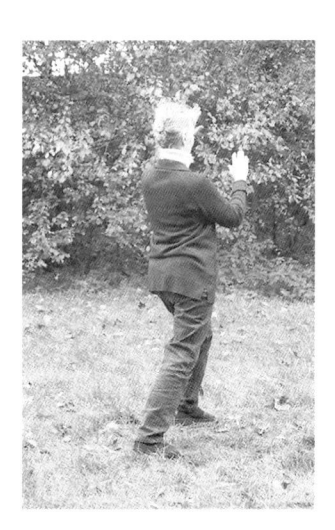

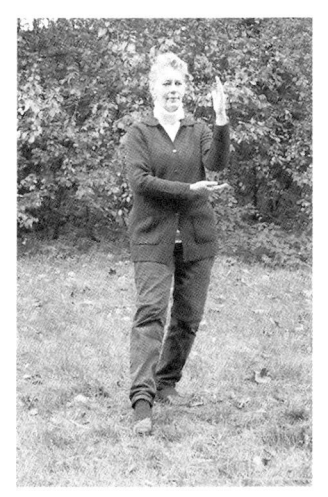

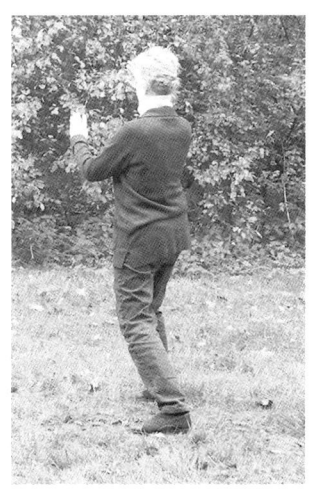

109

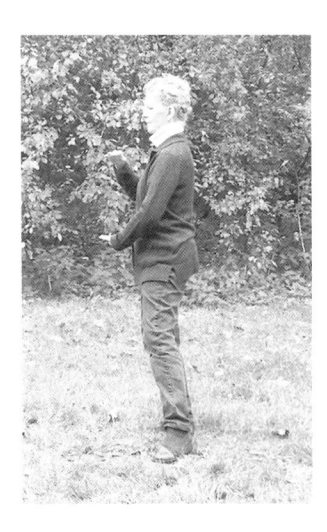

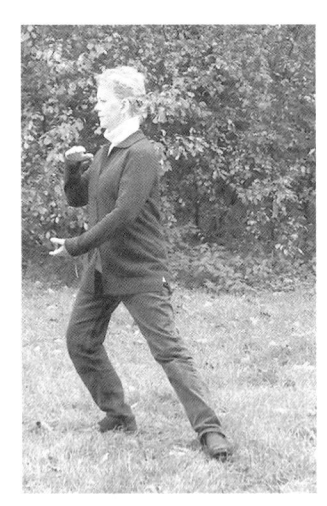

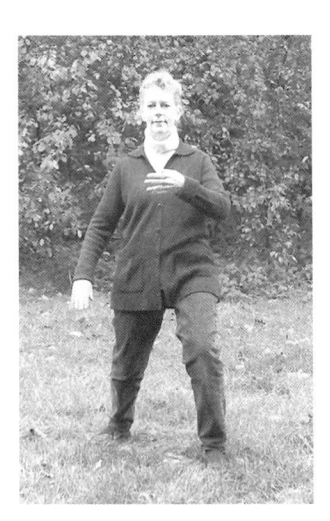

GRASP THE SPARROW'S TAIL WARD OFF LEFT

Shift all the weight into the right foot as the body turns to the east. Left foot turns on the ball, both hands come down, left palm under right as if holding a beach ball, step out widely with left heal, as you shift weight into the left leg, left hand rises, right hand comes down. When over 50% of your weight is in the left foot turn the hips to straight, the right toes turn in at a 45° angle. The finished posture is left palm facing the chest, the right hand down by your right side in front. 70% of the weight is in the left leg, 30% in the right. Body facing north.

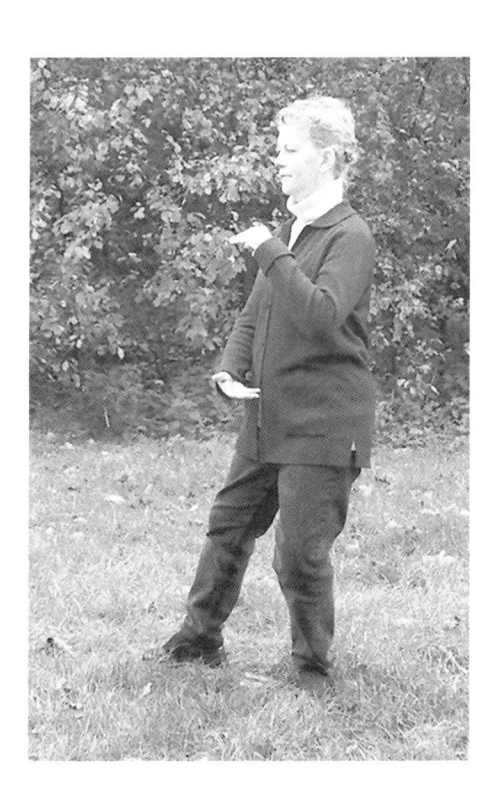

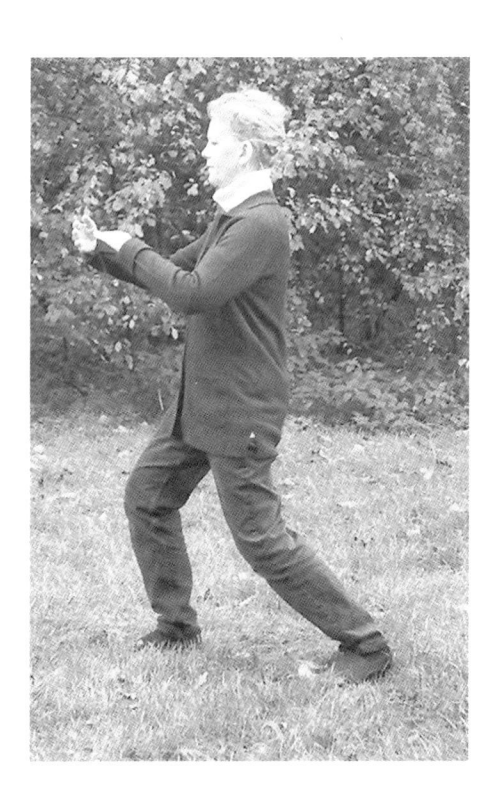

GRASP THE SPARROW'S TAIL WARD OFF RIGHT

Shift all the weight into the left foot as you turn on the ball of the right foot. Bring the right palm underneath the left, as if holding a beach ball. Step out widely onto the right heel. Shift weight into the right foot as the right hand rises to chest height, the left fingers pointing at right palm. Turn hips to the right facing east, the left toes turn in at a 45° angle, 70% of weight in front foot, body facing east.

GRASP THE SPARROW'S TAIL ROLL BACK

Turn your waist to the right 10°, keeping the weight distribution the same. Sit back onto your left leg. As you turn, the left hand comes down round and up in an arc of a circle to ear height, while the right hand comes in front of your body. All your weight is in your left foot.

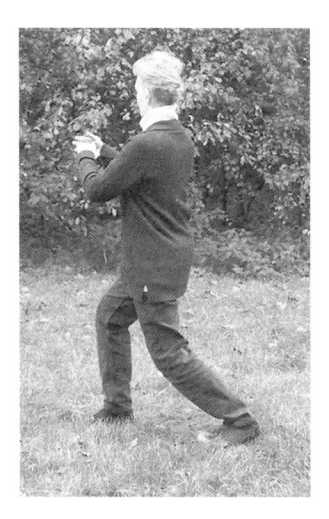

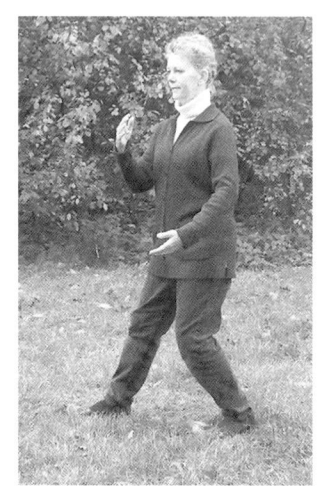

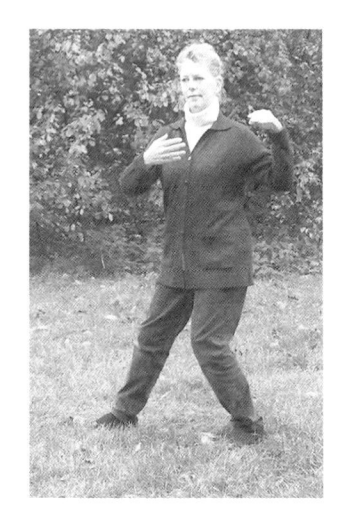

GRASP THE SPARROW'S TAIL PRESS

Shift weight back into the right foot as the left palm comes forward to touch the right inner wrist, chest height, hips straight. 70% of weight in right foot.

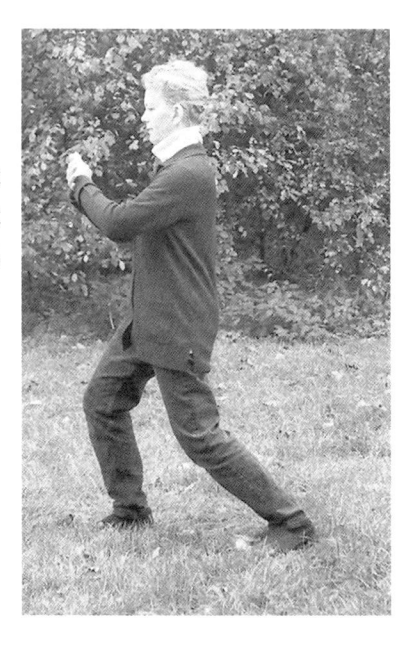

GRASP THE SPARROW'S TAIL PUSH

Sit back onto the left leg, hands separate, shift into your right leg, push with the hands, fingertips shoulder height and chest width, elbows bent. 70% of your weight on the front leg.

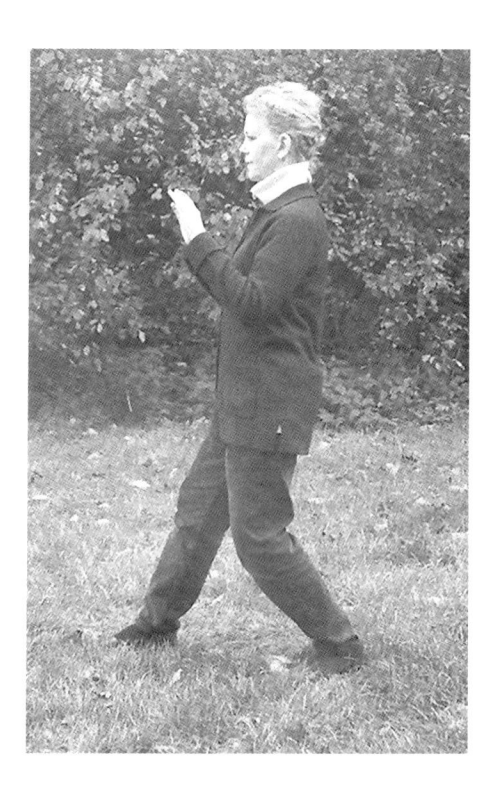

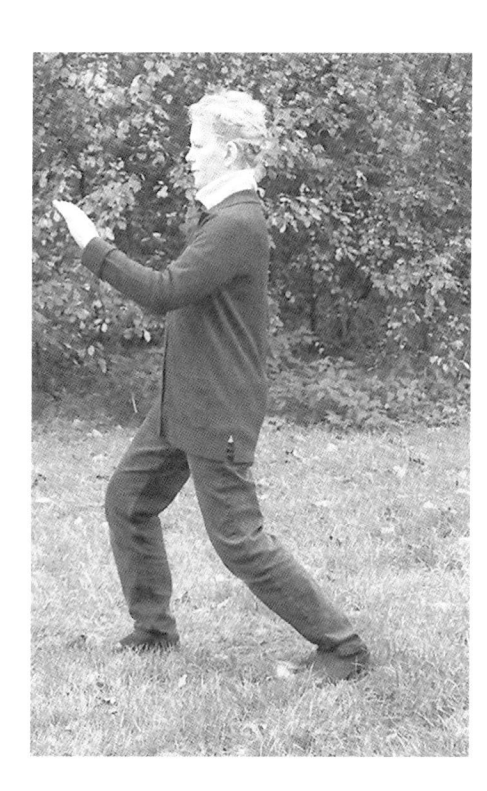

SINGLE WHIP

Sit back onto your left leg, the arms come down parallel to the ground, elbows slightly bent, all the weight is in your left leg. Turn your torso and the right toes to the left as far as they will go, your nose, navel and arms maintaining the same relationship to each other. Shift the weight back into the right foot as you turn the waist to the right. Left hand comes down with the palm facing up underneath the right hand, all the fingers of which are joined in the shape of a bird's beak. All the weight is on your right foot. Turn the hips to the left and pivot on the ball of the left foot, the right hand formed as a beak moves out to the corner, shoulder height. Step out widely onto your left heel. Shift the weight into the left foot, the left hand rises in front of you, turn your waist to the west, the right toes turn in at an angle of 45°, at the last moment the left palm turns over.

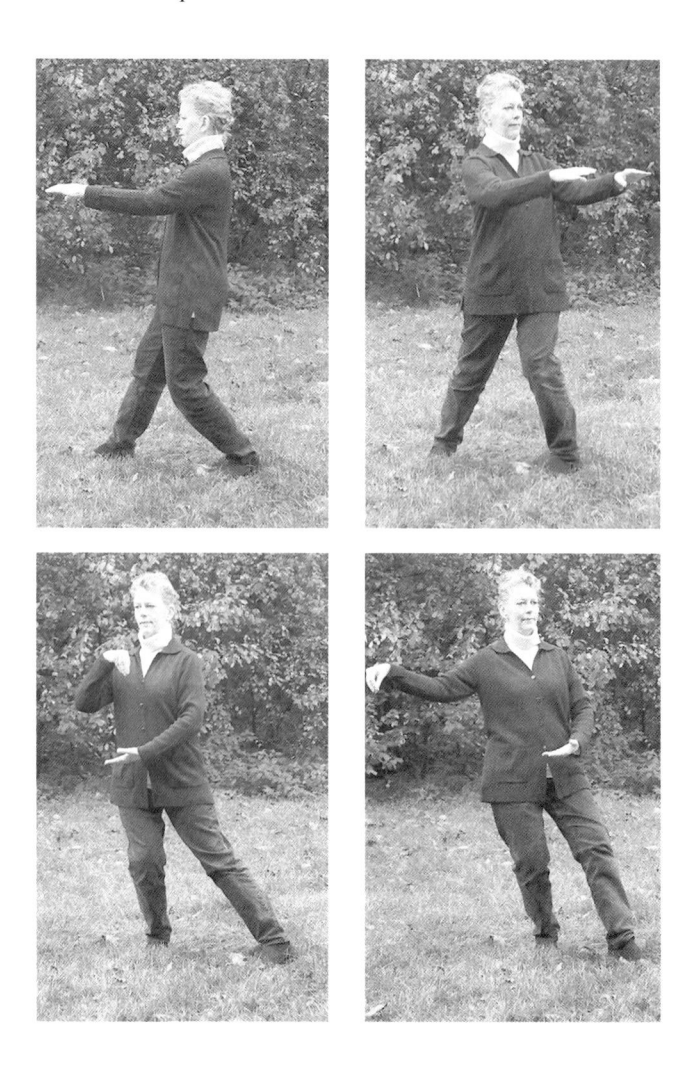

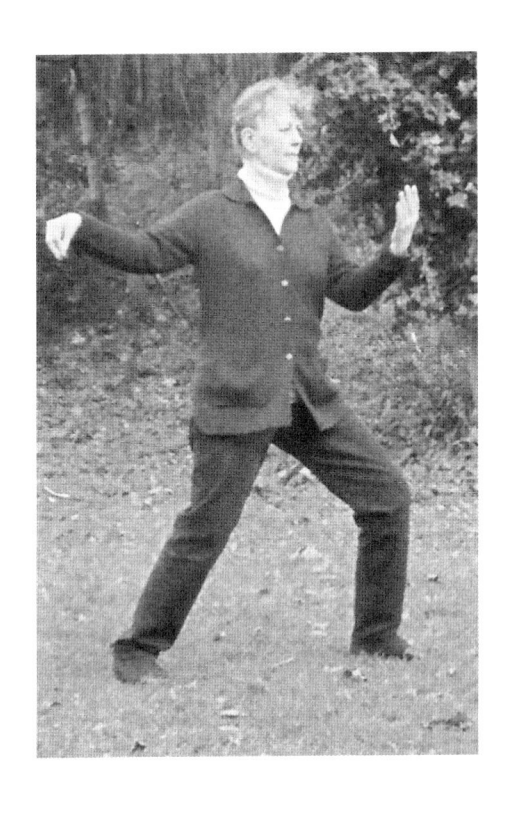

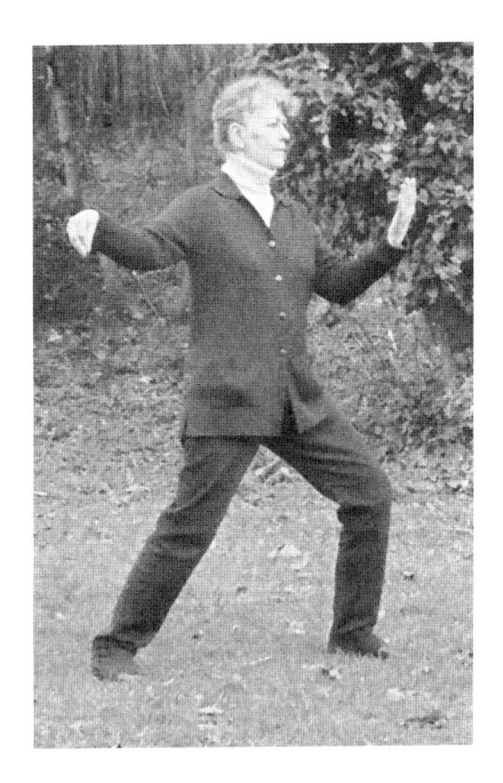

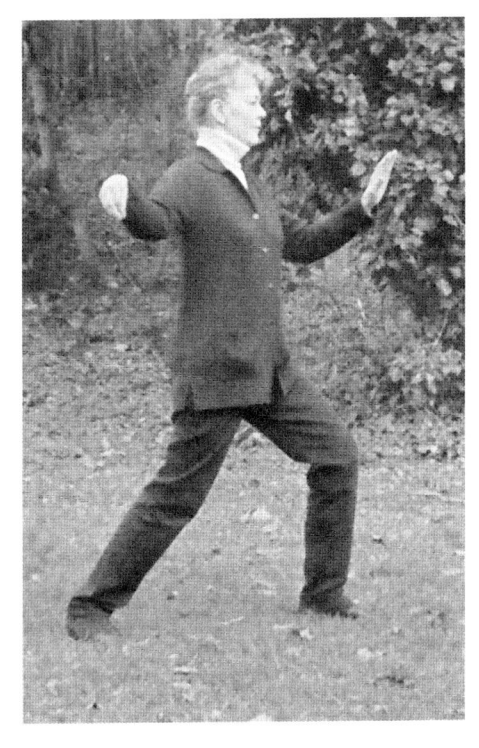

SNAKE CREEPS DOWN - SQUAT SINGLE WHIP

Turn to the right, as the right toes and left palm turn to the right. Sit back and sink for the Snake Creeps Down. The left hand comes back slightly, fingers pointing forward, turn the left toes in 45°. As you shift the weight into the left foot the left hand moves forward on the inside of the left thigh. Left toes turn out 90° to the corner.

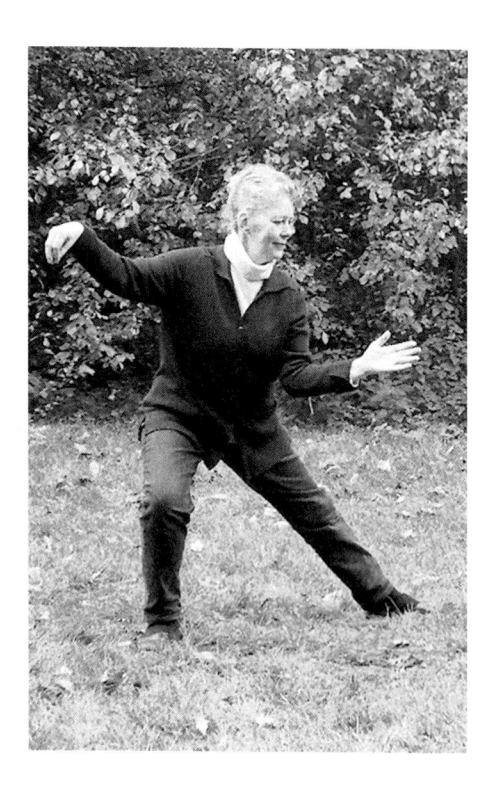

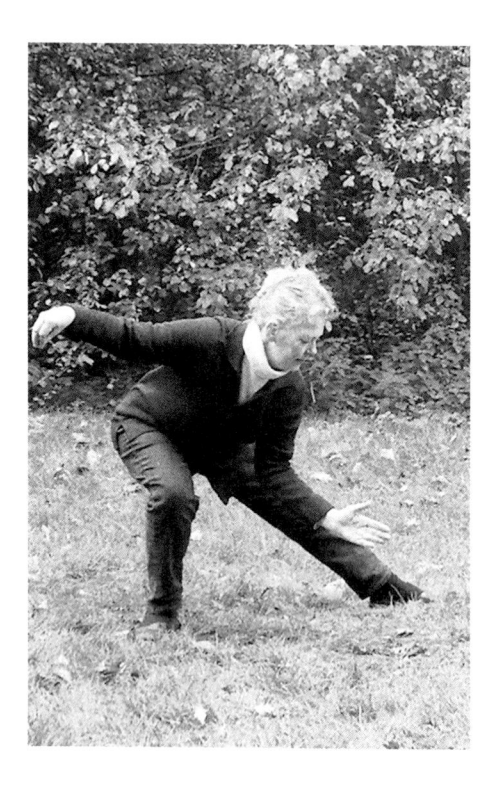

STEP FORWARD TO THE SEVEN STARS OF THE DIPPER

When around 70% weight is in left foot, right toes have come in 45°. Left hand moves up to above navel height as beak comes down to behind right thigh. As you come up onto your left leg, The right foot steps forward weightlessly and rests on the ball of the foot in front of the left, simultaneously the beak opens as the right hand comes up in front of the body re-forming into a fist at the same time as the left hand forms a fist, both joining in a block, just below the wrists. Neck height with right fist in front of left, body facing west.

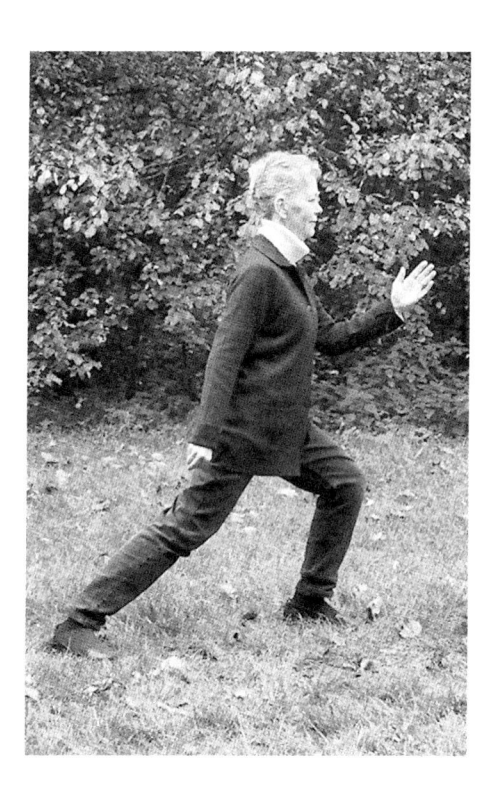

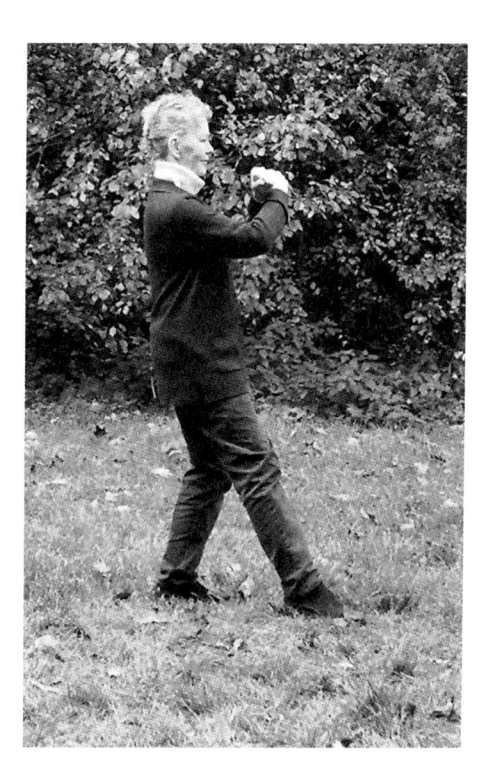

STEP BACK TO RIDE THE TIGER

All the weight is in the left leg. Step back onto the right foot ball first. Shift weight into the right foot, hips begin to turn to the right, simultaneously both arms come down, fists open, hands separate, so when all the weight is in the back leg the body is facing north, northwest. Right hand is near right thigh, while the left hand is in front of navel. As the hips turn to the left, the right hand comes up by the right side fingers pointing straight up as the left hand brushes knee, while the left foot sweeps to the right, all the weight in the right foot.

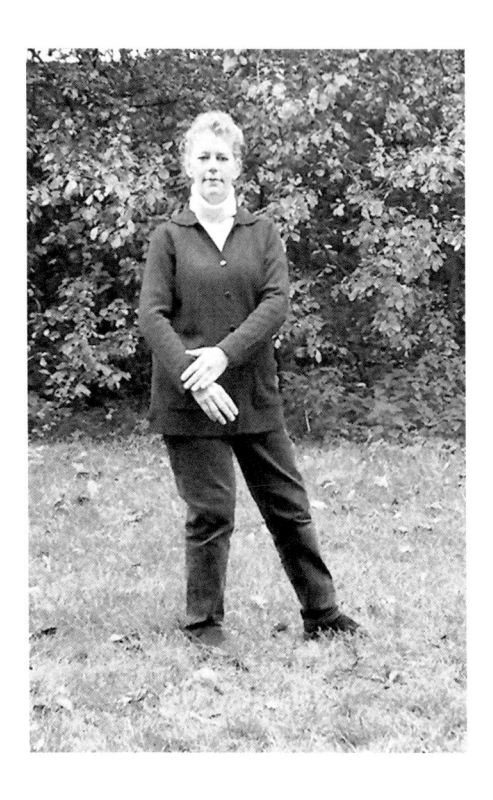

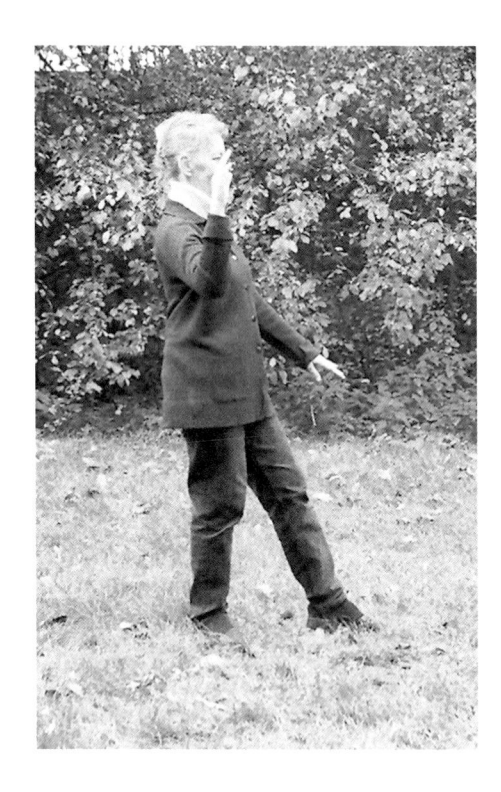

TURN BODY AND SWEEP LOTUS WITH LEG (LOTUS KICK)

Turn torso to the left while right arm comes down, both arms move to the left in a circular configuration. Swing and pivot round on the ball of your right foot propelled by your left arm and left leg in a circle, landing on the heel of your left foot behind the right leg, facing southeast, continuing the circle on the heel of the left and the ball of of the right foot until you face west, 100% weight in left leg, both arms are now facing forward, parallel to ground, elbows bent. Execute Lotus Kick. The right foot turns to left, circles up and kicks fingers of both hands, then comes back towards the left leg without touching the ground, and steps to northwest, heel first.

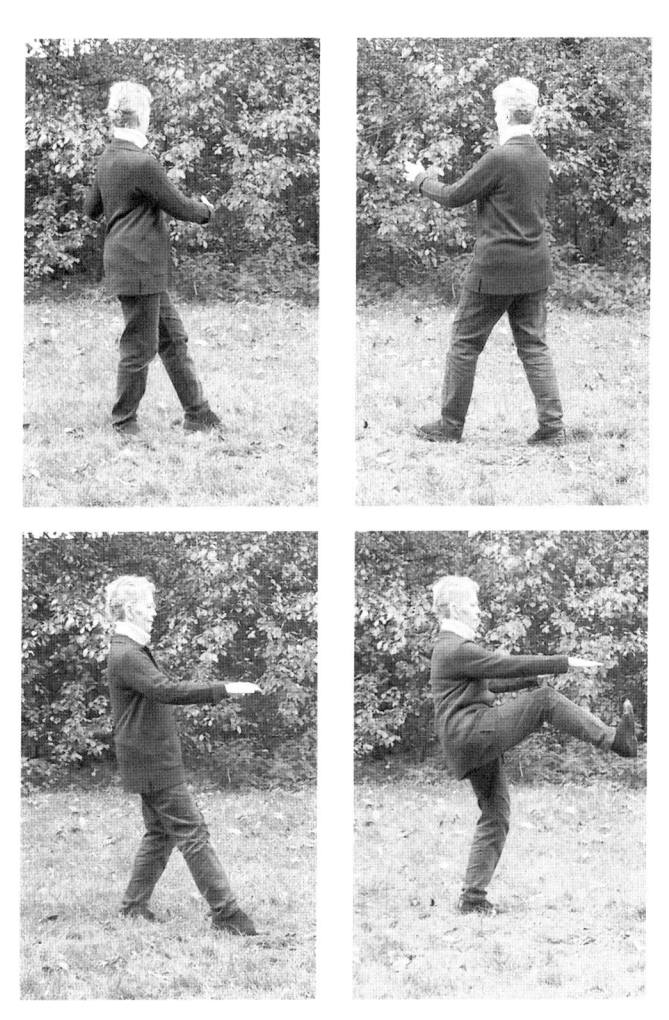

BEND THE BOW TO SHOOT THE TIGER

As weight shifts into the right foot the hands come down to just below navel height, as the hips turn to the right, hands rise up forming fists to head height, right higher than left. As the hips turn to the left to point to west, right fist strikes at head height, as the hips then turn to the right to face northwest left fist strikes straight in front of you. 70% weight in right leg.

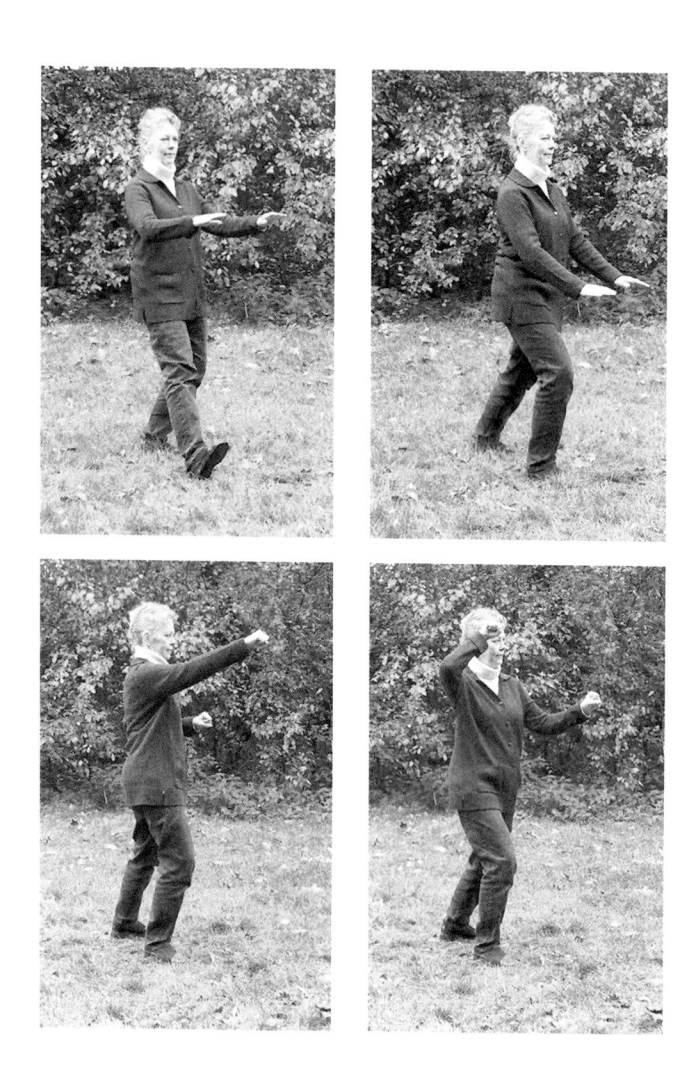

STEP FORWARD, DEFLECT DOWNWARD, INTERCEPT AND PUNCH

Shift all weight into the right leg, lift left foot, replace, shift weight back into left leg, torso turns to the left as both hands come down with left fist opening, right remaining by navel. Step to the northwest corner with the right foot, hands come round in front of you, left palm in front, right fist by your right hip. Left foot comes forward, shoulder width. Body facing northwest. As you shift the weight into the left foot the right fist comes forward in an arc, then a straight line as you strike with the fist, while the left hand comes down and back to behind right wrist, 70% weight in the left foot.

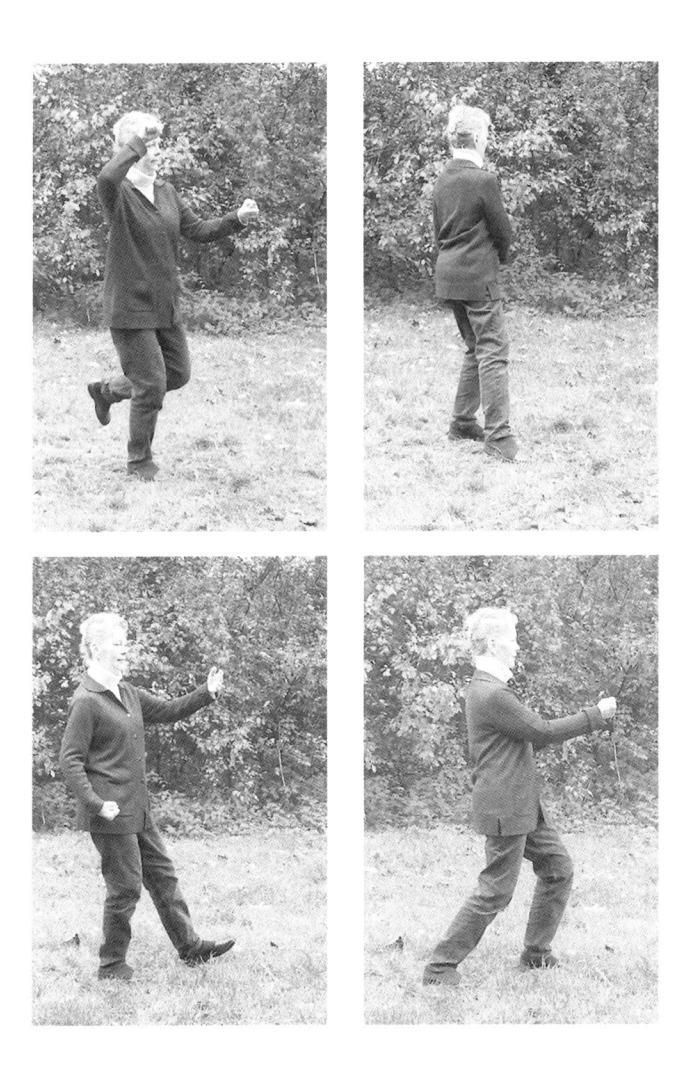

WITHDRAW AND PUSH

Keeping the weight distribution the same turn the hips to the left, the right hand opens as the arm extends. Turn the hips back as you sit onto the right foot as the right hand passes through the left elbow joint. All the weight is now in your right leg. Shift weight forward into left foot, push with the hands, chest height and chest width, until 70% of your weight is in the front leg.

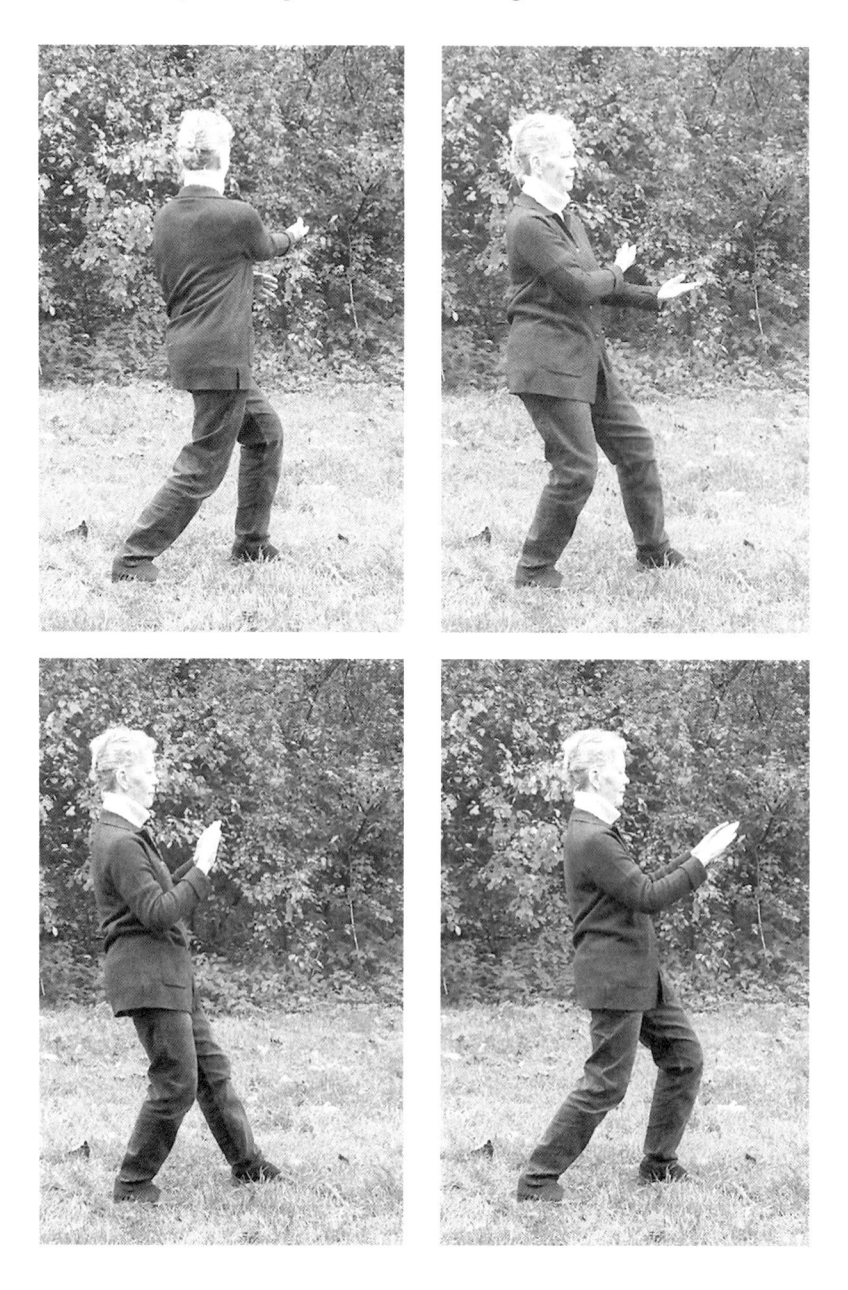

Side view from the Punch

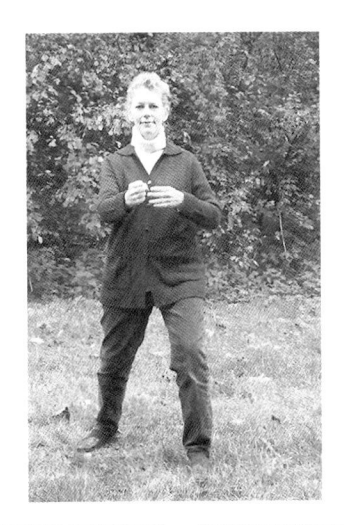

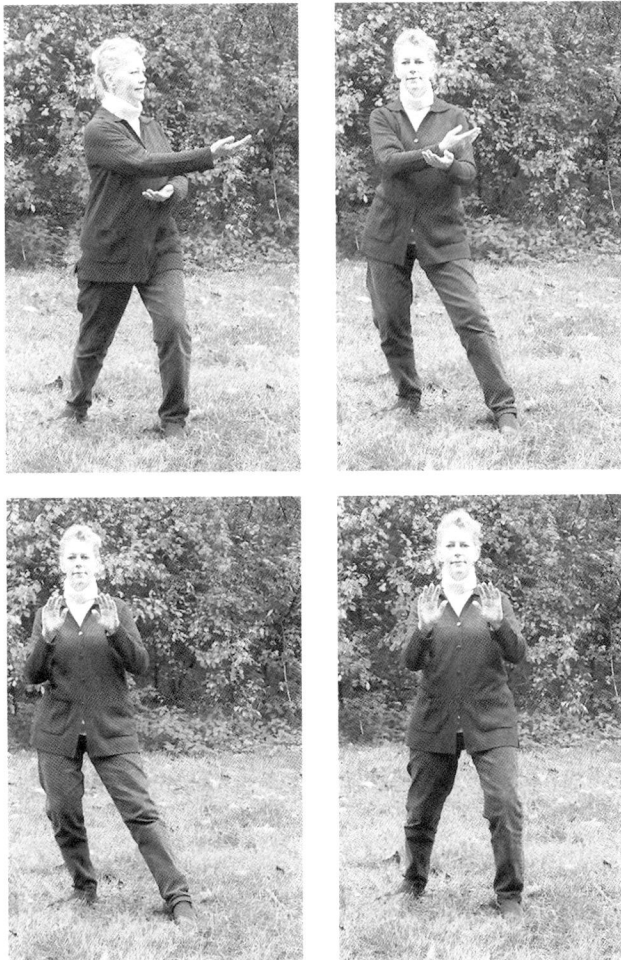

CROSSING HANDS

Sit back onto your right leg as you turn to the right, right hand circles out as you turn your left toes 90°. Shift all the weight onto the left foot as you turn on the ball of the right, the left hand goes out and down in a circle, right foot steps back in line with left as the arms come round in a circle and meet at the wrists, chest height, right in front of left, palms facing body, crossing at wrists. Weight evenly distributed in both feet.

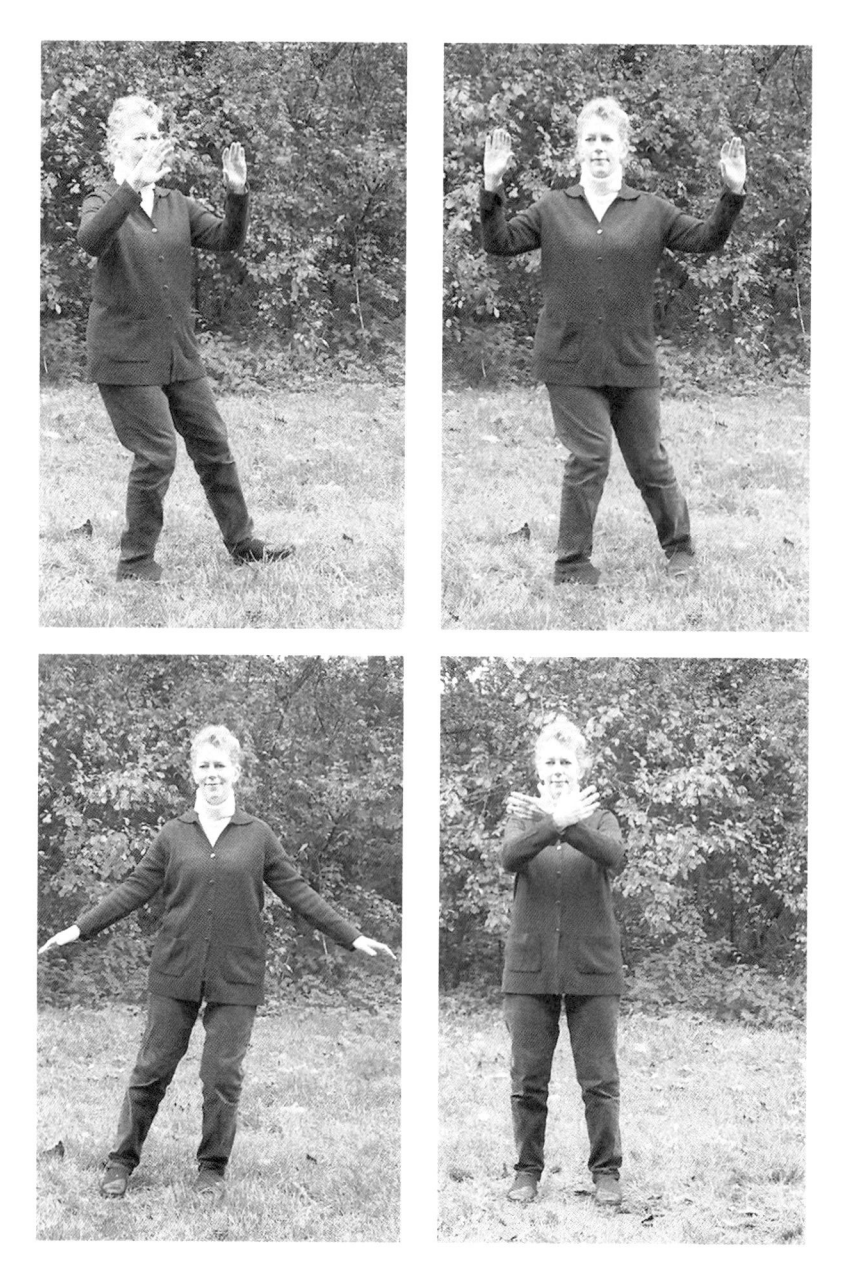

CONCLUSION

As you stand up erect without locking your knees the hands come down by your sides, palms facing backwards.

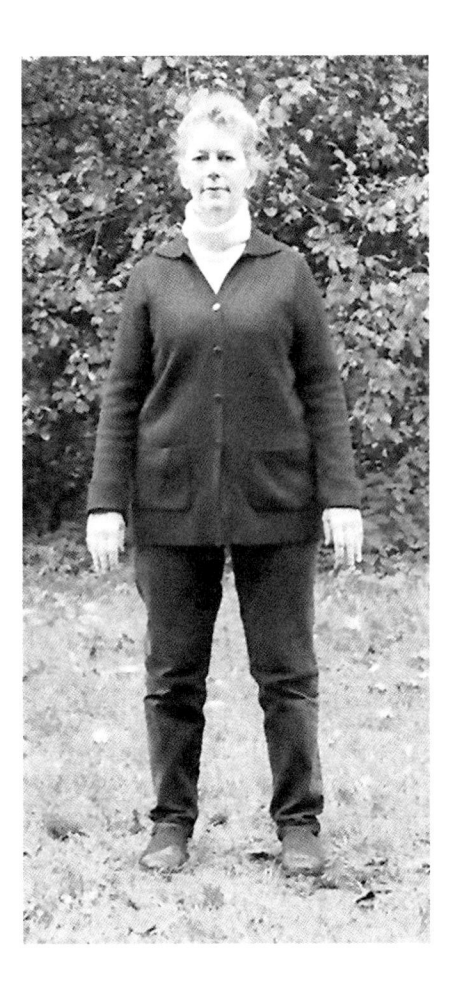

SECTION FOUR

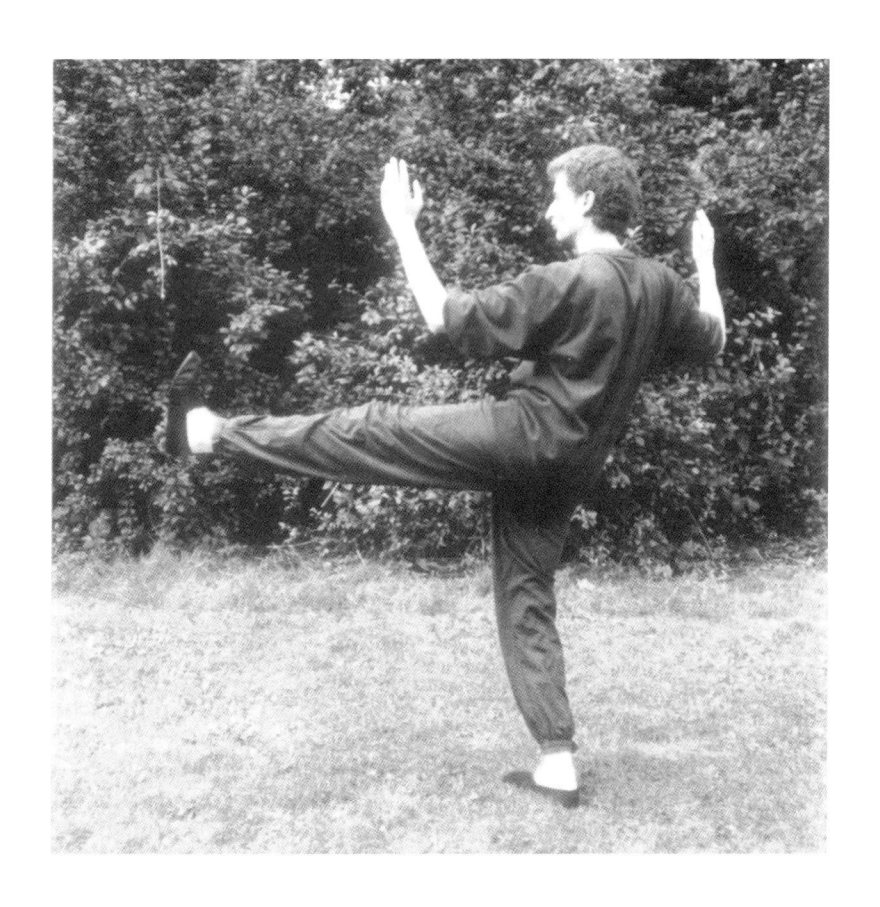

More on Exercise

Clinical studies in China confirm that a combination of callisthenic exercises practised in conjunction with T'ai chi and Chi Kung compounds their benefits. Callisthenic exercises primarily improve the condition of the skeletal muscles, while T'ai chi and Chi Kung serve to improve the function and condition of the internal organs. Healthful exercises, as we have seen, are moderate and continuous in nature and are practised over fairly long periods of time. Fitness exercises are more energetic and are practised vigorously for a period of time in order to increase heart rate and consumption of oxygen.

Without regular exercise it is harder to maintain fitness. The more you use your body the fitter you will become. Health and fitness are separate phenomena. Health being defined as freedom from disease and fitness relates to our ability to meet the demands of the environment. Components of fitness are: muscular strength, muscular endurance, cardiovascular endurance and general flexibility. Muscular strength, flexibility and stamina are maintained by regular use. Strength training requires that muscles be used at more than 80% of their maximum strength for short lengths of time, with the demands being increased periodically. Cardiovascular exercises are any exercises or activities that stimulate the heart and lungs for a period of time; often they are done for up to 20 minutes at a time.

Healing exercises build physical strength and improve physiological functioning. By improving our strength and increasing our body's ability to resist illness we are less susceptible to the effects of external factors. Our reserves of energy are increased by exercising on a regular basis which improves the function of the immune system. Loss of vitality could be due to under use and under stimulation of the various vital functions. Staying healthy may depend on regularly exercising the body.

Without daily exercise it is difficult to stay fit. Everyone should keep up a reasonable level of fitness. Adequate physical activity will help one deal with the stresses of modern life. Regular exercise can be the means to an alert, vigorous and healthy life. The old Chinese proverb 'running water never goes bad' could be taken to mean that the human body will remain in good condition as long as it is exercised on a regular basis.

Quality of Life

There is no doubt that by exercising one feels better. The effect can be therapeutic as structured, organised demands are placed on the body. There may be a positive psychological change as people begin to feel better about themselves. They may even look better. Their ability to concentrate may improve as well as their will power becoming stronger. As the condition of their body improves, they are more prepared to meet the demands of everyday life.

To recap - physical training makes the heart work harder and beat faster. This results in lowering the heart rate when the body is at rest. Increased circulation provides muscles with the necessary supplies of food and oxygen. A strong efficient heart pumps more blood with less effort, enabling one over time to exercise for longer periods. Regularly exercising the major muscle groups increases the size of the muscle fibres; this helps pump more blood to the heart. This is why it is important to maintain muscular strength into advancing years.

Advancing Years

If people, as they get older, reduce their activity and minimise their exercise, their tendons and muscles will shorten, causing stiffness in the joints. The ability to twist, bend and turn will be limited. Reduced muscular development will result in lower reserves of strength, which could result in strained muscles and ligaments. It is said that sedentary people may have slightly thicker blood, which does not flow so well. Any aerobic activity (walking, swimming, cycling) if practised daily or several times a week will make the heart work more efficiently as it becomes more resilient.

The body and its functions adjust in relation to the demands placed on them. Diminishing the load reduces muscular strength. The heart becomes weaker and less efficient, the body becomes less capable of meeting physical demands. Inactivity leads to weakness - there is decreased flexibility in the joints and the lungs become less efficient.

Age is no barrier to maintaining fitness and wellbeing. By exercising, one may be slowing down the aging process as the body parts are kept clean and well lubricated with increased blood circulation. An aging body will respond well to moderate exercise demands. Moderate exercise can be maintained for longer periods without fatigue. Gentle rhythmic movements such as in Chi Kung and T'ai chi, when practised regularly, can maintain and restore the full range of movements in joints, as well as increase muscle strength and improve endurance, capacity and stamina. These exercises may be the means to an alert, vigorous and lengthy healthy life. When practised consistently they will encourage joints to be more flexible, ligaments to be more elastic and muscles to become stronger. Being fitter and healthier will enable one to get more out of life in many ways.

Reasons for Exercising

There are many theories that attempt to explain people's behaviour. As human beings we are complex organisms, needing satisfaction, nourishment and challenges. Each person is different, unique and totally individual. We all share some similar behaviours and tendencies.

Some individuals are attracted to exercise as an 'aesthetic experience'. One of my closest friends was drawn to study T'ai chi when she saw a T'ai chi practitioner perform his T'ai chi form. She thought it was one of the most beautiful things she had seen.

When I enquire in my T'ai chi classes why students exercise, they generally say it is for health and fitness. They want to improve their overall wellbeing. They exercise to feel better physically and psychologically as well as to relax.

Many people have an inner drive. They aspire to the goals they want to achieve. They generally want to be healthy, look good, have plenty of strength and fitness in order to get on with their everyday lives.

Some will exercise because they see themselves as potentially vulnerable. Their motivation for action is driven by conflict. Their action is designed to reduce the conflict, which was initially created by their fear of some potentially negative consequence.

Many adults frequent gyms to lose weight - they exercise because they feel so uncomfortable with how they look. Their actions are designed to comfort their minds more than to exercise their bodies. Their actions are not necessarily designed to achieve something but to get rid of something.

Some individuals exercise for the social experience, in order to increase their circle of friends and perhaps to find like-minded people to interact with.

Benefits of T'ai chi and Chi Kung

An effect of attending T'ai chi and Chi Kung classes is that one's health and fitness improves. Having exercised, students feel the benefits. They then reason that it is important to continue the process. Through persistent training, they notice an overall change in their minds and bodies. They feel and may look different; other people may begin to respond to them in a new way. Their life changes through the medium of exercise. This can lead to more interest in self-development. Their thirst for knowledge grows, as well as perhaps the need to satisfy some inner urge. Sometimes people come to classes in order to release tension and pent-up emotions. For many people the stresses of everyday life seem to be increasing. Many do not have ways of releasing this build up of stress. Very often they just suffer.

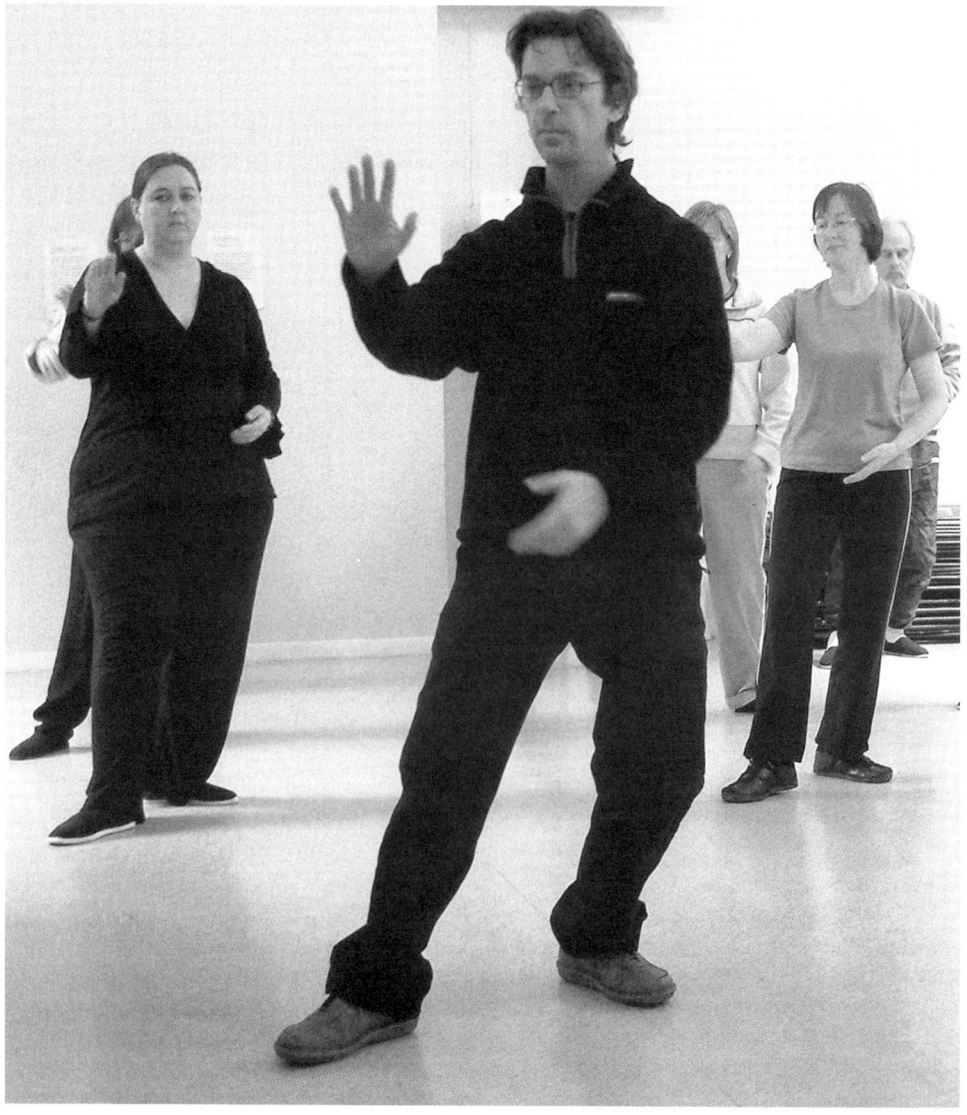

No Exercise

If exercise is so important why do so many people not exercise on a regular basis? People come up with all kinds of reasons for their inactivity. Some possibilities may be external factors such as time, opportunity, dependence on the co-operation of others and lack of facilities.

Others justify not exercising using reasons such as tiredness, lack of will power or motivation. It is important that these people realise that the demands of society may gradually increase over time. If people's minds and bodies are not increasing in capacity and strength, then these demands may exceed their ability to cope, which may result in all kinds of uncomfortable conditions. Cheng Man-Ch'ing was of the opinion that people are generally lazy. If this is true, then one can conclude that the application of will may be necessary when the flesh is weak.

Adult Education

All kinds of exercise classes are now appearing in Adult Education. There is so much interest and demand that the classes fill up very quickly, often with waiting lists.

Being in a class situation can trigger all kinds of responses in students. Some enjoy it, some resist slightly, some try and control as much as possible, while others end up needing to be pampered. Students come into the learning situation with certain attitudes, perceptions and expectations. Some have specific needs, desires and aspirations. A proportion of them may have low self-esteem, arrogant behavior and issues over control and authority. The teacher has to be able to collate all of these factors as well as prepare and execute information in an instructive, easy to understand manner. Having done this, the teacher needs to encourage, lead and inspire the students to do their own work to reach their desired objectives.

The Teacher's Perspective

In a teaching situation it is important to understand motivation and how it can affect a student's progress. It is why a person is taking this action, the reason for doing this specific thing. Some know why they do what they do, while others may not be quite so clear in their thinking. When a person knows what they want, and why they want it and by when they want it, then they are more likely to be able to make calculated decisions about strategic actions they are going to take to achieve their goal by the deadline.

Any action can be taken for several reasons. The action may in itself be the goal. It may also be the process by which one achieves one's goal. Generally, action is taken to go towards something or to go away from something. Action is motivated by either desire or conflict. If by desire, the motivation comes from within and is freely chosen. If the driving force is conflict, then obligation and circumstances other than free choice dictate the action taken. Conflict driven action may work short term but it is difficult to maintain and sustain momentum over long periods of time.

Teachers need to encourage their students to go for their aspirations and goals without manipulating them in any way to achieve this. The teacher is sometimes the students' motivator, gradually encouraging them to motivate themselves. As a facilitator you are leading them where they want to go, showing them the quickest route to the desired outcome, enabling them to learn what they want to learn as soon as possible.

The Learner's Role

Once on the learning journey some students get disillusioned as a result of the class being harder, easier or different to what they expected. Also the time factor comes into play. They want results sooner than it may be happening. They may then get to a critical point where they lose interest, enthusiasm and energy. Often at this point they drop out of a class. Persistence and patience are two important points to always keep in mind. One's initial enthusiasm may wane over time. Sometimes the teacher's enthusiasm is enough to get students beyond this point but really the students have to address their own thinking as this is ultimately what is going to lead to continuation and success. If students lose sight of their goal, they may temporarily get distracted by current difficulties or inability. This may lead to feelings of mental as well as physical discomfort. When teaching, one has to always remind the students where they are going in case they veer off course.

The T'ai Chi Learning Environment

In my experience of teaching T'ai chi, people of all ages and abilities attend the classes. The speed of progress is generally set by the slower students. I find I have to be aware of the more able students so as to keep their enthusiasm and momentum going. I have to evaluate constantly the progress of the class and sometimes adjust and change my plans.

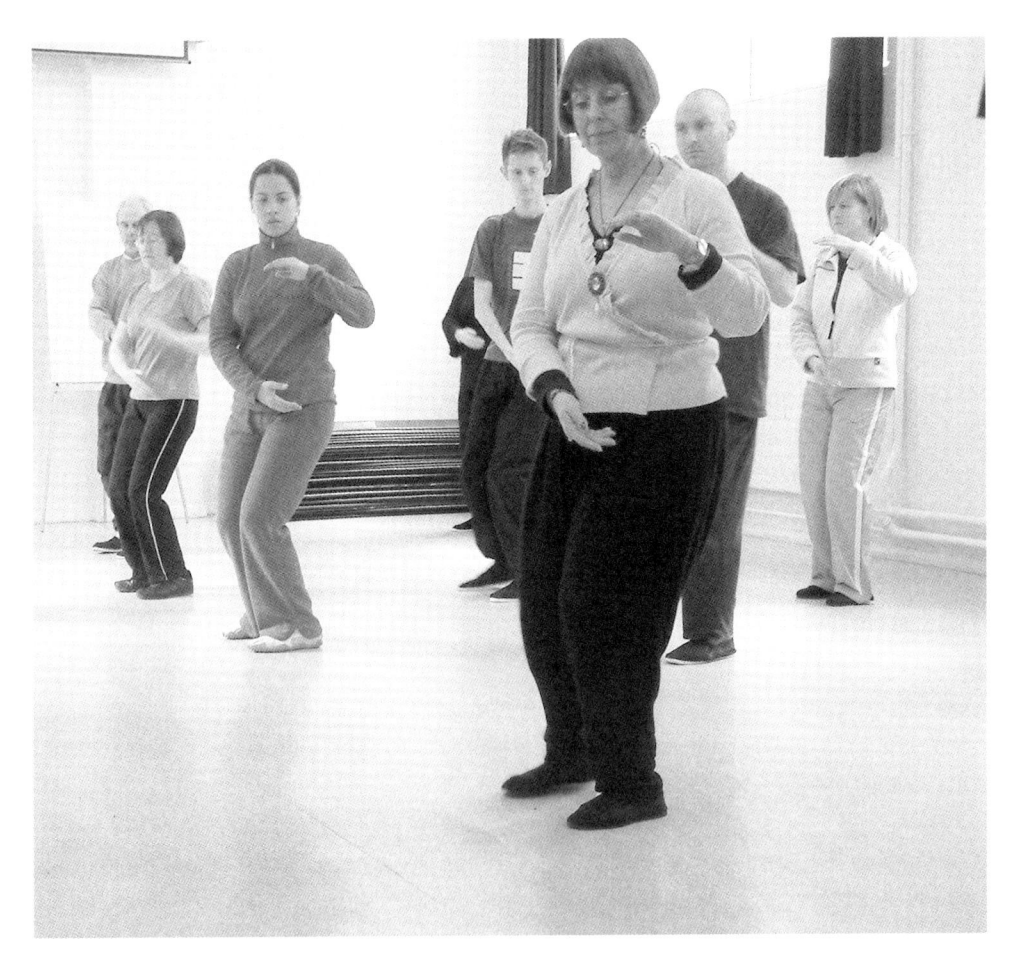

The students' learning environment has to be friendly, nourishing and humorous. Sometimes if people take things too seriously their attitude can interfere with their capacity as they become associated with what they do. This can create an emotional burden, which can add even more complexity to the difficulty of their task. Once a more light-hearted humorous approach has been created, then I find their relationship with their own learning improves. They are able to separate themselves from what they are doing in such a way that it does not reflect on them.

The amount of practice that a student does at home greatly affects what can be achieved in the class. In T'ai chi the general overall capacity and progress of the whole class can be hindered by those who do not practise because the whole class does the movements together. When the majority of the students in class train at home, then even the ones that do not practise improve as if carried by the work of the others. Those who do not practise will have to rely on the other students. When in the class, they are able to perform but when out of class they are lost.

A student with great potential who does not practise will not be able to do the movements well. As a teacher, there is nothing one can do to make the student do the work. You can instruct, show, guide, inspire, but if they do not do the work they will not have the capacity, irrespective of their aptitude and ability.

Those students who do practise need to be nurtured and guided in the right direction. The importance of practice needs to be emphasised. Without correct consistent practice, progress may be erratic and slow. Becoming responsible for their own learning will lead to progress. In certain oriental approaches, the teacher is seen as a signpost showing the way and it is the students' job to take action consistent with the directions. The more action taken, the further they will go. If enough time is spent on the path, they will reach their destination.

The Teacher's Role

From a philosophical point one can ask which is more important - being on the path or reaching the destination? People differ in opinion about this point. As a teacher, you are hopefully guiding students onto their most appropriate path, encouraging them to constantly travel further along it so that they can learn more and more from their experiences.

The teacher has a responsibility to use a wide variety of teaching methods. The approaches need to be broad enough to encourage interest and enthusiasm in the students for the subject, irrespective of their starting point. Sometimes people come to the class with learning difficulties. Others may have physical disabilities. In these specific cases, more teacher time may have to be spent with individual students, constantly encouraging them to build on what they currently have. Whatever a student's level, it is important to praise their current efforts, as you work with their strengths, develop their areas of weakness and add to their existing knowledge base.

Over the years, I have studied accelerated learning techniques where great importance is placed on exercising the various mental capacities. There are a great number of exercises to develop people's visual, auditory and kinetic functions. Generally people may have one faculty which is more dominant that the others. Some people may be more left brain oriented while others are right brain. Research has shown that by developing both sides of the brain simultaneously, one may be accessing more of one's potential. In my teaching I use visualisation as a way of developing the right side of the brain. In the oriental approach to teaching, it is quite normal to answer a question with a story. Somewhere in the story is the answer.

Even in the western approach to learning, the use of the right side of the brain is encouraged because thinking pictorially may help intelligence, due to the fact that one is thinking dimensionally rather than linearly.

A teacher's task, irrespective of who is in the class is to:

- prepare information
- deliver information
- explain about the information
- inspire the students to want to learn the information
- guide the student's assimilation of the information
- encourage the students to learn for themselves from the information
- guide the students to search for more information to expand their capacity and potential for future learning

Personality and Character

People who are drawn to the T'ai chi class have a certain nature. Those whose personality does not suit this discipline eventually leave. Our personality and character can affect what we do and how we do it. From an early age we are absorbing information from many sources. We learn from watching our family, friends and others in our environment. We are born with certain tendencies, aptitudes and potentialities. We are drawn to certain things and sometimes it is as if certain people and situations are drawn to us.

As a teacher it is important to observe your students' personalities and characteristics, in order that your perception and understanding can lead to helping them maximise their learning. They come to you a certain way. Your task is to utilise what they already have in order to make the most of their current capacity, developing it in the most appropriate direction.

Personality and Character - What are they?

In the dictionary, personality is defined as the sum total of all the behavioural and mental characteristics by means of which an individual is recognized as being unique. Character is defined as the combination of traits and qualities distinguishing the individual nature of a person or thing.

Personality is generally seen as a good thing. If you are seen as having a lot of personality, people more often than not will respond well to you. Some people are not always complimentary about other people's personality as they focus on their most striking characteristic which they do not like (e.g. aggressiveness). How we respond to the world emerges from our personality, which is a combination of our character, temperament, intelligence and physiology. Psychologists are generally interested in the ways people differ from one another, as well as how the different aspects of the individual relate to each other. They are curious about the differences in perception and how these relate to the individual's total functioning. Generally they are looking at the ways people differ and what causes those differences.

Personality is the way we see ourselves and the way we are seen by others. Certain personality traits are perceived as more appropriate in various activities and situations. People's successes and failures sometimes are seen as being linked to their personalities. Personality appears to be a puzzle, purely because of its nature. Personality is something each of us is, and because of its mystery the best we can do is experience it.

Are we born with a certain personality or character?

It is generally acknowledged that children are born with certain potentialities. What happens to these potentialities depends on their experience whilst growing up. So it could be true to say that one's personality develops over time in relation to the environment we find ourselves in. Freud was of the opinion that what goes on in the family shapes the child's personality, especially in relation to human relationships. Each pattern of parental behaviour may affect the personality development of the child. The parents can be seen as role models to aspire to, or the child may react against certain parental tendencies. Theorists claim that children learn roles appropriate to their sex, ethnicity, age, family, class and religion. Society and culture bestow on them identity, personality and a feeling of self.

We are born into societies that are already organised into roles and these show us what is expected of us. Children learn this quickly. Adult behaviour also conforms to social roles. Human behaviour is malleable and easily altered by the environment, which may shape our motives, desires and wishes. We create our environment from our thinking and the environment we create helps to condition us.

Teaching

A teacher needs to be able to interpret a student's personality. Not only that, the teacher needs to be able to encourage students to expand, develop and express their capacities. Irrespective of the teacher's personality, he/she should be able to relate to the student's personality. Learners need to feel encouraged to participate. From a learning standpoint the teacher's personality is important. Research shows that effective teachers are firm, kind and demanding.

Rosenshine and Furst found that the following teaching behaviour helps learners to learn:

- Being clear
- Being enthusiastic
- Using a variety of approaches
- Good questioning
- Being task oriented
- Being indirect (giving clues so that the students learn independently)
- Giving learners an opportunity to learn
- Making structuring comments

Liking the teacher is important for student success. The teacher needs to know the subject well, making it easily digestible for the students. The teacher's competence affects the student's effectiveness.

The pupils need to be stimulated to want to learn, having had their interest aroused, as well as having their curiosity and intellectual capacity excited. They may want their emotional needs met by the teacher. This will be achieved when they feel safe and secure in the class, and when they find the relationship with the teacher rewarding.

These days a teacher's task is not just simply imparting information but also transmitting values and attitudes. The teacher is now becoming a counsellor, psychologist and friend. This is why teaching is such a challenging task. The ability to deal with each person's individuality in class in such a way that it affects all the personalities in the class is especially an art.

Understanding human nature is important, so that our individual nature does not interfere with our capacity to learn and grow. In T'ai chi this capacity to understand human nature comes from our own journey into our personality. We begin to discover how we work. In the Chinese approach there is a belief that each of us is a microcosm of the universe. In order to understand the universe, we need to work on understanding ourselves. In looking at our own learning capacity and process, we can gain insight into other people's capacity.

There is a saying; 'You are what you think, having become what you thought.' We are led to believe, based on this statement, that all the thoughts we have ever had in the past have encouraged us to be how we are now. This statement of course does not take into consideration that our past experiences in our environment also influence us. Nevertheless for now let's look at this statement.

If one adheres to the thoughts of the past, then one's future will closely resemble one's past. If our thinking in the present differs from the past, our future will be going in a different direction to what it would have been, if our thoughts had stayed the same. Our thoughts affect the course of action we take; the action we take gives us direct feedback about the effectiveness of our actions. This feedback will either confirm that our thinking was correct or it will encourage us to change our thinking for the purpose of advancement and learning. People sometimes get attached to particular thoughts or ways of thinking - this sometimes gets in the way of their learning.

What we currently think may at some point influence our future. The now is influenced by our past thoughts. If we think the right thoughts, in the right way, then we encourage and heighten the probability of the right things happening.

Certain personality types may think in certain ways; how appropriate their thinking is depends on the task at hand. If the task is learning, then the teacher will see if their current way of thinking is speeding their progress on, or slowing them down.

Learning

Learning is the absorption of information which was previously unknown, by means of assimilation. Through the application of the now learnt knowledge, a deeper understanding of the information will be acquired which, over time, will become even deeper. A feeling of knowing will be experienced at a certain point as a result of applying the information.

The willingness of a person to take on new information without knowing how true it is, shows their openness and willingness to learn as well as showing their trust in the teacher and the process. Some people are receptive to the unknown, whilst others are carefully sceptical. There is an art to learning and absorbing information. Many people interfere with the absorbing phase of learning by trying intellectually to fit new information into their current database, before it has had a chance to be digested and sorted out naturally.

Sotto (1997) confirms this by saying:

> *We do not have to do anything in order to understand. All we have to do is come to that which is to be understood with an open mind, to immerse ourselves by degrees in it, to be patient, and to allow the situation to unfold itself. After that comes the need to check whether what we think we have understood corresponds to reality.*

Certain aspects of personality are positively related to success in learning. There are three important aspects:

1. Intellectual ability
2. Personality types
3. Motivation

Intellectual Ability

It can be assumed that some people are born more intelligent than others. These people can be described as luckier, as they have more inherent potential for success in any endeavour. Irrespective of one's current level of intelligence, it is good to know that learning can be affected by proper training and tuition. Our current capacity is only our starting point; it is the foundation on which we will grow. We may or may not start with an aptitude for a particular subject, but with correct tuition, work on our part, and given sufficient time, we will be able to achieve our goals if it is within our genetic capacity.

A determining factor in relation to intelligence is genetics. It affects our temperament, however it is not as visible in relation to our values, ideals and beliefs. Temperament can be perceived by looking, for example, at people's energy levels when active and at their emotional levels when interacting with others. Genetics really give us our individual uniqueness. Psychologists suggest that our emotions are innate, having already been coded into our genes. So choose your parents wisely!

Intelligent teachers are also going to be potentially more effective teachers, as this enables them to discern facts about their students more easily, enabling them to interact appropriately with their students, encouraging good teacher/pupil relationships.

Teacher's Observations

I find that people of varying ages, from differing backgrounds and environments come to my T'ai chi classes. They show different levels of ability and I find it interesting to see that their progress in learning T'ai chi may sometimes be improved by their intelligence and sometimes hindered by it.

I remember as a T'ai chi student being told by my teacher in a class that we were all too intelligent and it was interfering with our T'ai chi progress. How can this be so if intelligence is an aspect of personality that is positively related to success in learning?

One could say that intelligence is how quickly one comprehends and understands. This differs from ability, which is the capacity to act wisely and effectively on the thing comprehended. So intelligence does not necessarily mean success. It is the ability to apply what has been comprehended which gives capacity and eventually success.

I notice in T'ai chi classes that it is the intellectually oriented people that sometimes have the most difficulty. I have concluded, over the years, that this is due to the fact that they have left brain dominance. Their linear intelligence capacity is excellent but their right brain, spatial and dimensional capacity is less developed, thus accounting for their difficulty in class. My teacher's suggestion for us to be dumber, may actually be just a different way of saying that we should use our left brain less, thus encouraging both sides to work equally, so as to enhance both of their capacities.

Much classroom education these days is a case of feeding the left brain more and more information. We are encouraged to think, analyse and dissect things. This may end up being detrimental in the application of right brain activities.

Personality Types

The two most recognised types of personality are extroverts and introverts. It is generally agreed that introverts study better as their focus generally is inward, they have more practice at being focused on one thing. Extroverts are more focused outwardly. They are often more energetic and sometimes more emotional. In the learning process it is useful to listen and be quiet; extroverts may find this harder. No one is totally one of these types as people display varying degrees of each at various times.

I come across introverts and extroverts in the T'ai chi classes I teach. My job as a teacher is to work with people's diverse personalities in a way that encourages them to experience varying possibilities as a result of their learning.

Motivation

Some individuals are driven to achieve, to create, while others find it harder to muster up the enthusiasm and energy to do what is needed. In the teaching role you have to be willing at times to be the less motivated students' motivator. Your hope is that your enthusiasm and energy will trigger off their own enthusiasm. The drive that is generated in some people is the desire to achieve purely for its own sake, while in others it is a drive that may be generated by conflicts within the individual, where they feel the need to have to achieve. As a teacher you are guiding students' thoughts and actions, using the energy of their motivation as well as your own energy.

People do things for various reasons - for pleasure, for growth, so as to realise their potential, to understand things - they have a need to know. Motivation is the process that leads an individual to attempt to satisfy some need or desire. This in turn creates a drive, which energises behaviour. They then engage in appropriate activity in an attempt to satisfy their need/desire.

The need could be biological (e.g. thirst), it could be a need for stimulation, it could be a desire to paint a painting. Maslow realized that there was a hierarchy to people's needs. In order of dominance; they are physiological satisfaction, safety, love, self esteem and self actualisation. He also added the desire for knowledge and understanding.

A teacher's task is to arouse in the student the desire for participation in a learning process. Once that is achieved it is then a case of sustaining the student's enthusiasm for learning. One of the best ways to achieve this is by exercising the student's abilities to visualise and then aspire to the image. It has been said, 'You are limited by what you cannot imagine and what you will not aspire to'.

Anything that can create drive, enthusiasm and energy is the basis of intrinsic motivation in the class. The teacher is assisting the students to direct their energy.

Curzon (1996) mentions the effect of motivation in relation to instruction:

Motivation arouses, sustains and energises students; it assists in the direction of tasks; it is selective in that it helps to determine students' priorities; it assists in organising students' activities.

Push Hands

The art of push hands as practised by T'ai chi players is a sensitivity exercise to develop their ability to sense the intention of another person. It is a preset sequence of movements practised by two people. The aim is to disrupt one's partner's balance.

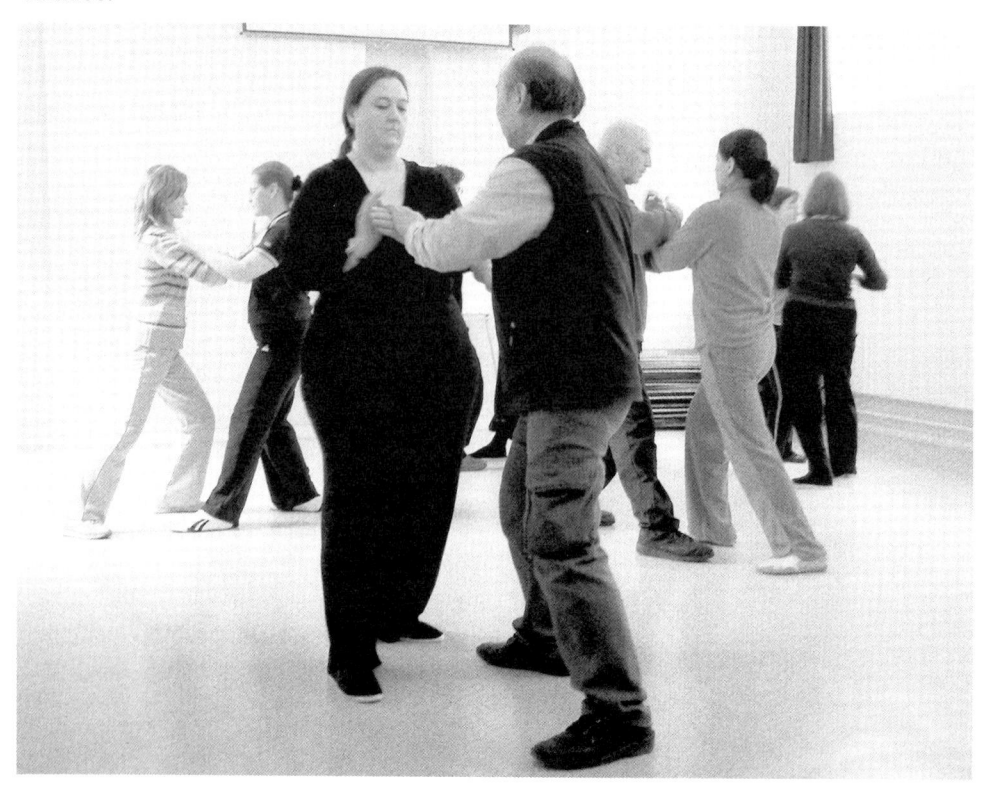

In ancient China push hands was used as a form of exercise to prepare students for the martial application of the T'ai chi form. These days push hands is generally practised for developing fluidity, mobility and alertness. Constant practice enables one to respond more efficiently to the actions of another person. With relaxation comes sensitivity, which enables the students to observe more with their hands. This usually leads to a deeper level of understanding of the art.

When doing the push hands form one becomes very aware of how appropriate or inappropriate one's actions are as one manoeuvres away and responds to the other person's potential push.

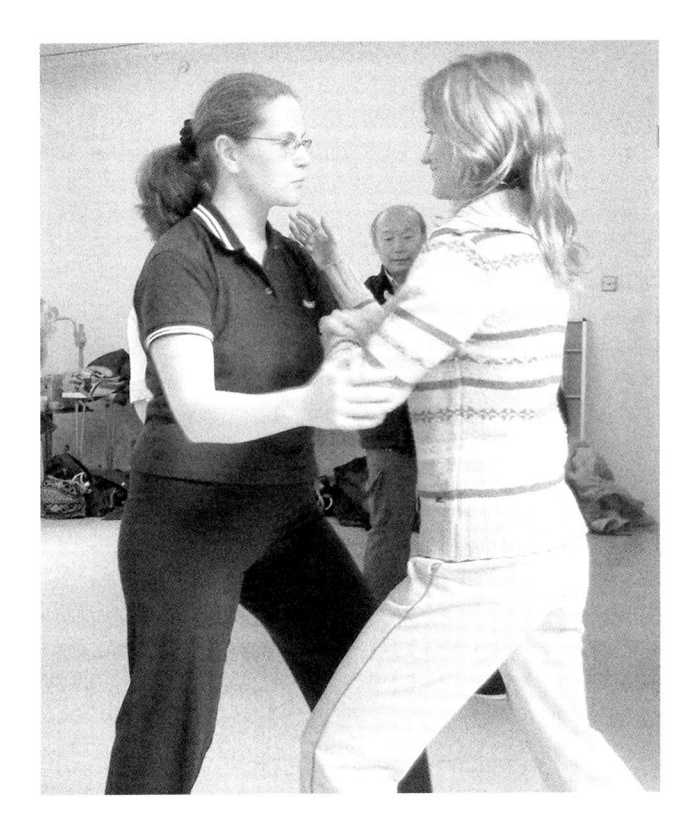

In T'ai chi we talk a lot about Yin and Yang and the balance of the opposites:

	Yin	**Yang**
	Quiet	Loud
	Dark	Light
	Inward	Outward

We see in the yin/yang symbol that at the extreme of yin is the beginning of yang and vice versa. Each has a dot of the opposite in it, each aspect is related to the other.

In push hands practice students are encouraged to experiment with each of these qualities (yin and yang) and varying degrees of each. The exercises demonstrate how one can change one's nature at will to suit varying situations.

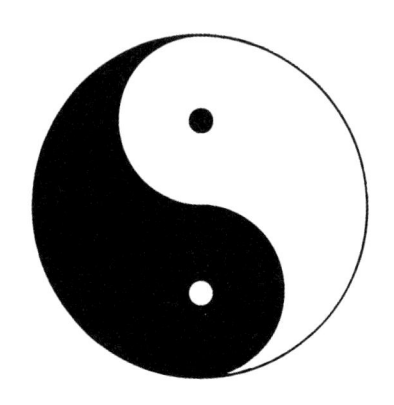

People's personalities have often taken a long time to develop. People also come in all shapes and sizes. Our physiques nevertheless do not determine specific personality characteristics but they may indirectly shape our personality by affecting how others treat us. In our enthusiasm to fit in and be accepted by our peers, we may take on certain characteristics, which are triggered off by other people's response to us. So we adjust our behaviour accordingly. It is good for students to see in a push hands class that they can choose consciously to be different and not have to respond in familiar habitual ways.

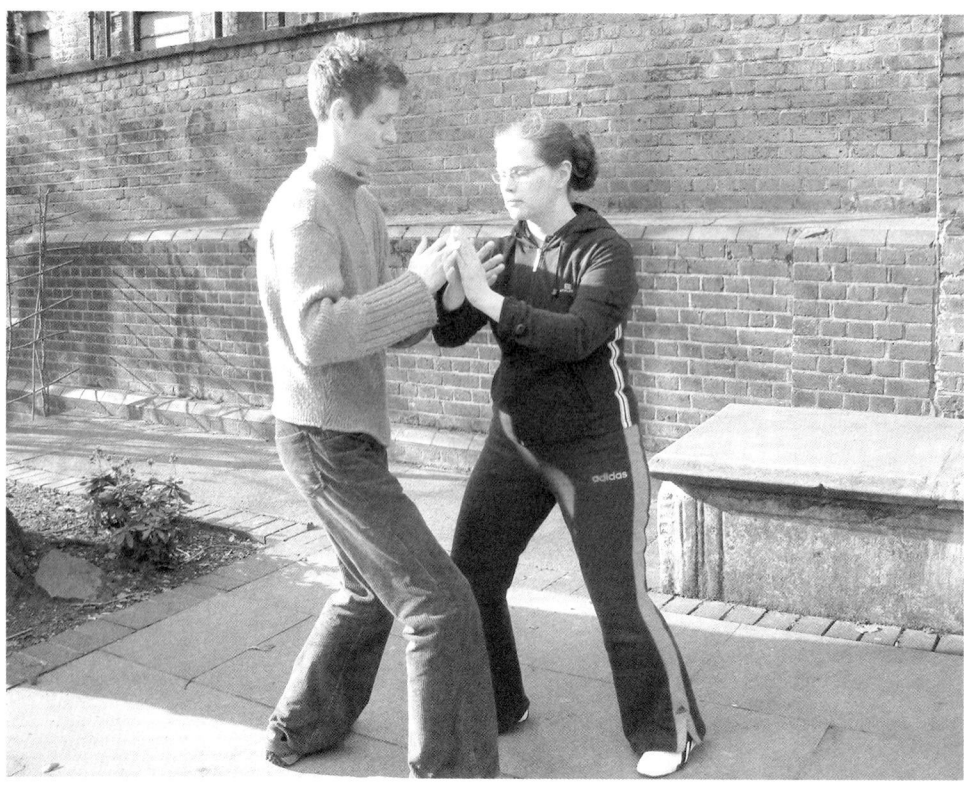

The push hands scenario is an opportunity to observe how your mind and body deal with pushing and being pushed. Some people do not like push hands as it brings out all kinds of emotions, feelings, reactions, memories, fears and aggressions. They may not have previously realised that this unique cocktail lay submerged below the surface of presumed calm and relaxation. What one observes at close quarters and in an intense way are life's principles, where there is a dynamic interplay between various forces at work in any given moment.

Often in everyday activities people react against circumstances or respond to circumstances, while others use the circumstances of their lives as the raw material on which to build. By being put in an intense push hands scenario, you begin to observe yourself and the way you operate as well as seeing how other people operate at close quarters.

Lack of mobility holds one back in push hands. Some people hold their ground physically and mentally. The emotion that fuels people's ideas and actions can lead to rigidity as they hold on in their bodies. In the push hands setting, any attachment to ideas and tensions prevents a person being able to respond efficiently to their partner's action.

'Invest in loss' and 'relax' are words I have heard hundreds of times in my own training. The word 'good' would come up when we were relaxed. Often we were admonished for being hard and tense. In push hands you are encouraged to let go, it is a gradual process that may be initially unsettling, confusing or even frightening to a new student. As you let go you interfere less with the process. You may end up developing what is known as 'economy of means' - thereby discovering more about simplicity as you develop your ability even further.

As you delve deeper into push hands practice, you learn more about yourself, especially your physical and mental constrictions. With time you may become calmer with yourself and others as your ability increases. It is often our own insecurities that make interacting with others difficult and complex. Understand yourself and you begin to understand others.

Your perceptions may be clear or confused; sometimes you have to work to remove the elements that create the confusion. When these elements are no longer in your life, situations become easier as you interfere less with yourself and others.

As a voyage of discovery, practising push hands is time well spent, as you learn more about yourself. Knowing more may make it easier to live with yourself, not to mention enabling you to interact and relate to other people more comfortably.

In the Class

Coming into a class situation people often bring with them preconceived ideas of what will happen, based on their expectations. If these expectations are not met exactly, some people become judgmental, dissatisfied and defensive. The teacher's role may be as a negotiator at this point to deal with people's perceptions based on their thinking.

In T'ai chi, part of a teacher's role is to encourage clarity of perception. This for some people is easier than for others - as some have a very strong conceptual view of reality, as opposed to seeing reality clearly as it is, without the colouring of their projections. Sometimes people have to go beyond the influence of their previous learning or incorrect learning before they can advance.

For many people image is crucial. In the T'ai chi tradition 'saving face' was of paramount importance especially in ancient China. Being seen a certain way and upholding that image was very important. These days students turn up to class with an image of themselves which they want to uphold. In a learning situation where something new is being learnt there are times when mistakes are made. This is a natural part of the learning process. Some people are not able to allow and tolerate mistakes on their part. They feel and think that it says something derogatory or negative about them. This attitude comes from a certain outlook on life which has now become an ideal for the person involved. They aim to live up to this ideal and sometimes if they do not succeed, they chastise themselves for their perceived failures. When teaching, one has to be constantly reminding students that it is perfectly permissible to make mistakes as this is a natural part of learning anything.

One projects onto one's future one's current thinking and the emotions behind those thoughts. Our thoughts precede our actions. We move in time and space into the manifestation of what we once thought. We experience the feelings that the emotions associated with the thoughts created. In reality we experience our personality in action. We go into what we have already set up for ourselves for the future. Each person sets up his or her future differently. Their chosen directions will either help them or not. When teaching it is important to teach and explain this above-mentioned point to students so that they can gauge how effective their current thinking is. This is extremely important in relation to self-image. Factors that influence our self image may be: our confidence level, our physical state, our energy levels, our self esteem, our previous learning and our learning capacity.

Our perceptions of ourselves are influencing our actions and behaviours as we attempt anything. When involved in learning new and complex subjects, we may find that our lack of ability and capacity may trigger in us negative preconceived impressions about ourselves related to our image and esteem. This can then interfere with our learning capacity, as we now begin to look at ourselves and how we are doing; we become distracted from our initial task which was learning.

Sotto (1997) wrote:

> *Some people have a dread of self-disclosure. Others find it difficult to assert themselves enough to take part in a discussion. Others have a poor self-image and stay silent for fear of saying something that might lower their self-esteem even more.*

It is important for the teacher to set realistic goals in the class, which are attainable. This will help students with their self-esteem. Once students have a good feeling about themselves based on their own progress and complimentary comments from their co-students, then the teacher and students have a good foundation for growth.

Brookfield (1986) states:

> *Those adults with positive self-concepts are thought to be more responsive to learning. Environments that reinforce the self-concepts of adults that are supportive of change, and that value the status of the learner will produce the greatest amount of learning.*

For learning to be successful we need good tuition, a modicum of ability on the part of the student, and practice in the form of work by the student using the information given by the teacher. Each student is unique and their learning will be most effective when their personal strengths and weaknesses are acknowledged and taken into account while teaching.

The teacher fills the gaps in their learning and provides the conditions that will enable the students to pick up the information in such a way that there is no waste of time or energy. The teacher is transmitting information, skills and understanding as well as awakening interests and encouraging creative thinking.

Handley states (1973):

> *It is the contact with lively minds that produces the thinking individual.*

Personality certainly influences learning for both student and teacher. As a teacher it is our role to be aware of differences and view them as a positive contribution to any classroom setting. In so far as a teacher's skill permits, sensitive guidance and awareness of individual characteristics and personalities is the foundation of a creative learning situation.

T'ai Chi Training

The T'ai chi curriculum may have changed over the centuries. Nevertheless certain components need to be in place for efficient results and effective training.

Students need to warm up and loosen up before being involved in any vigorous workout session. Moderate Chi Kung exercises are often sufficient warm up routines. Once the body has increased in temperature, it is then better prepared for greater challenges.

Meditation and relaxation exercises practised at the beginning of a work out session will help calm the mind and relax the body. The same techniques applied after a work out will help in the recovery stage, as healing and regeneration is facilitated. The mind is also brought back to a state of calm after the stimulation of the exercise.

Once sufficient warming and loosening up has been achieved, stretching exercises can be added to increase the range of movement at joint surfaces. Stretching will also help reduce the physical manifestation of tension. Undue muscular contraction if unchecked over time can lead to discomfort, pain or in some cases serious injury. There will also be a marked improvement in posture and alignment.

Chi Kung exercises will facilitate deeper levels of relaxation and higher energy levels. Consistent practice over time will increase strength in the legs, developing a solid foundation, which amplifies the effectiveness of the martial techniques.

The T'ai chi form is taught when a certain degree of flexibility has been achieved in the body. Other forms are added over time to increase capacity and understanding. The fast form develops increased levels of fitness, strength and flexibility. Working with a partner improves sensitivity and increases understanding of the practical application of the techniques. Partner exercises help develop flexibility and pliability as well as improving footwork. Weapon forms are taught to further increase strength, stamina and endurance. They also develop the practitioner's ability to project energy.

All these forms were originally developed as a means for self-defence. Knowing these different techniques generally increases confidence levels and can give great pleasure and enjoyment to the practitioner.

A student may not choose to practise or study all the different forms available; however any of the forms will help develop focus and attention. Practising these movements may improve the quality of life as well as help people realise their individual potential.

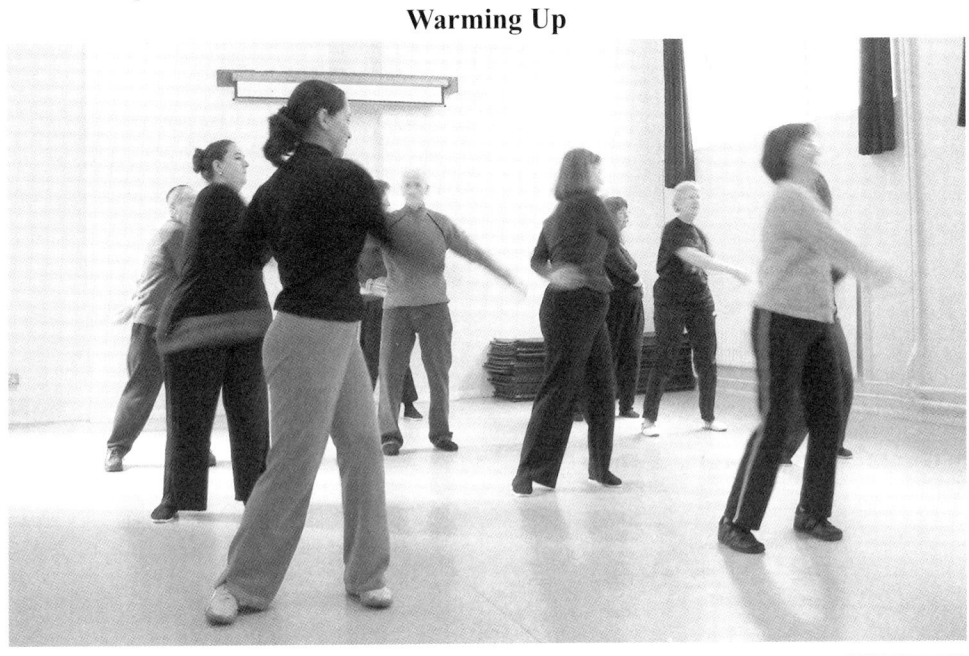

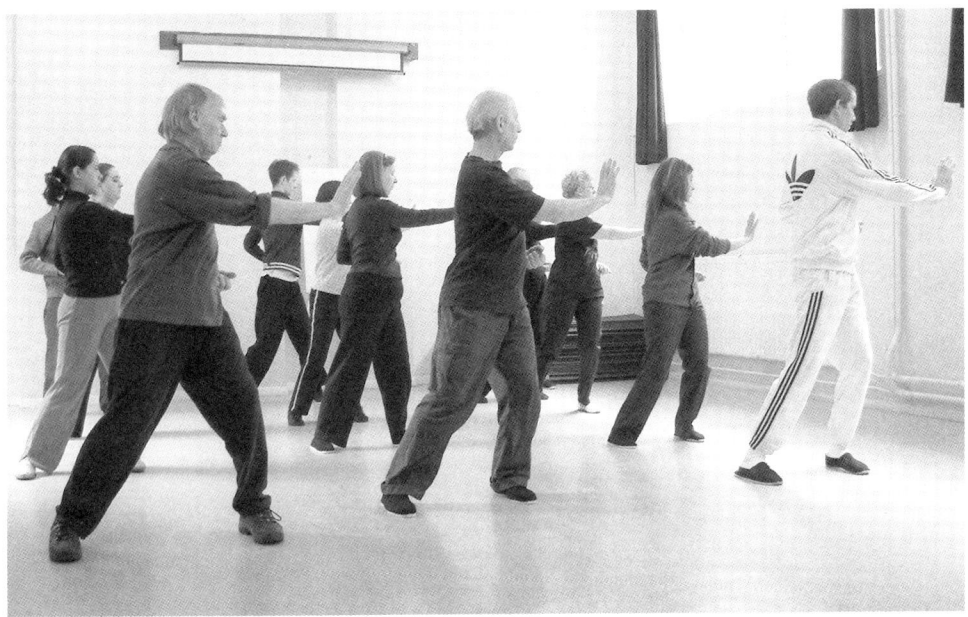

Warming Up

Stretching

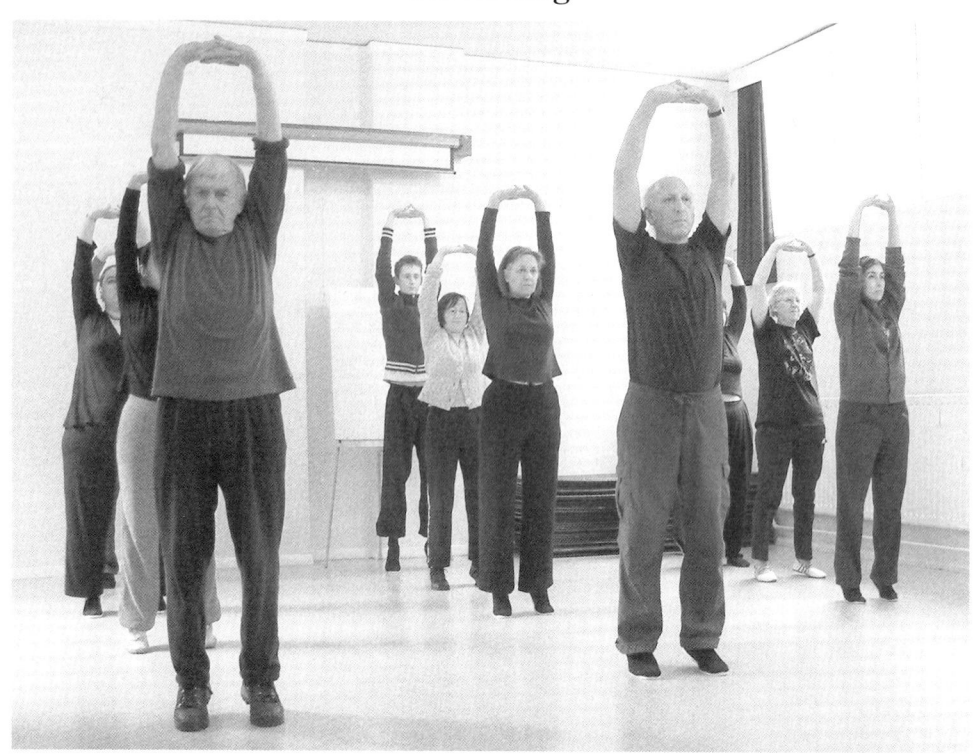

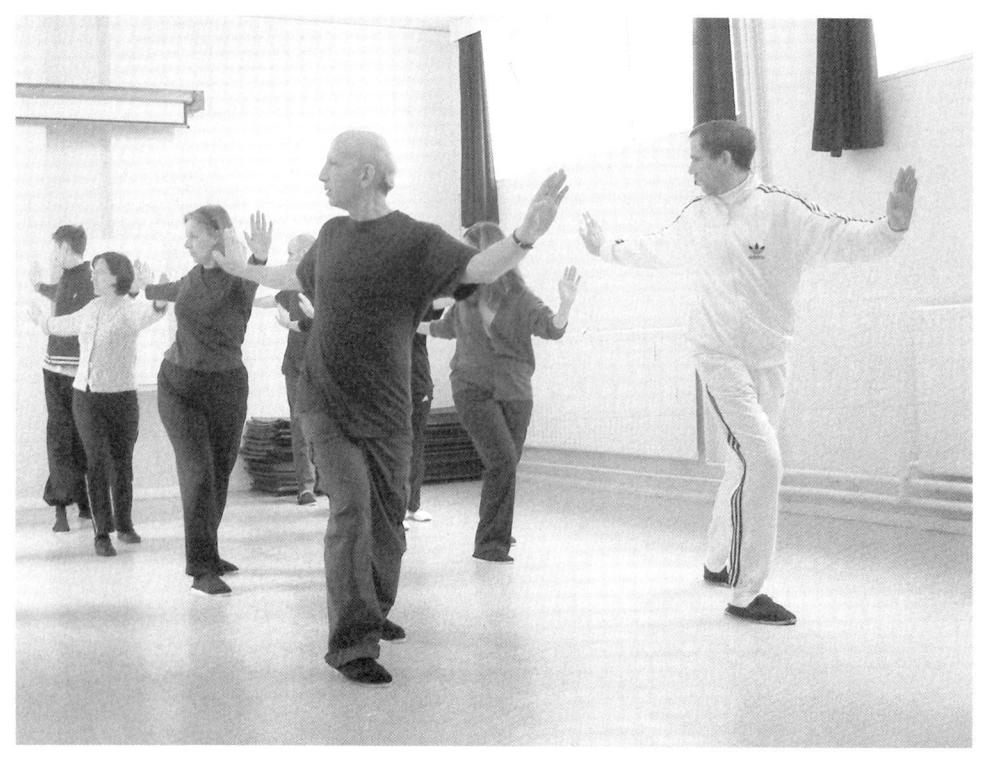

Chi Kung

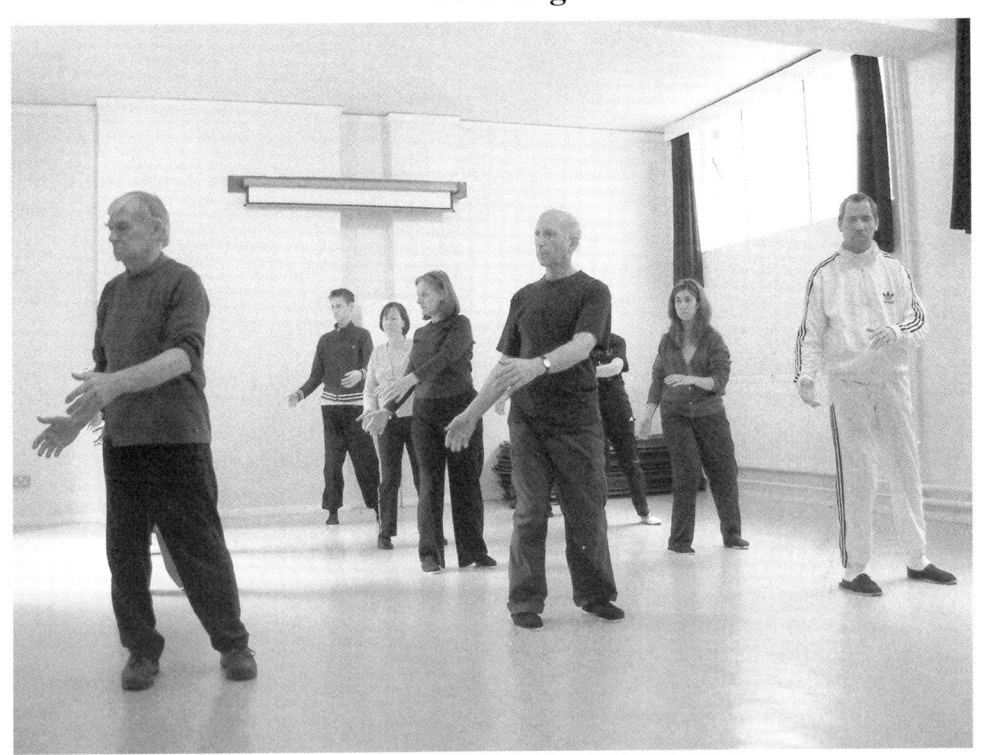

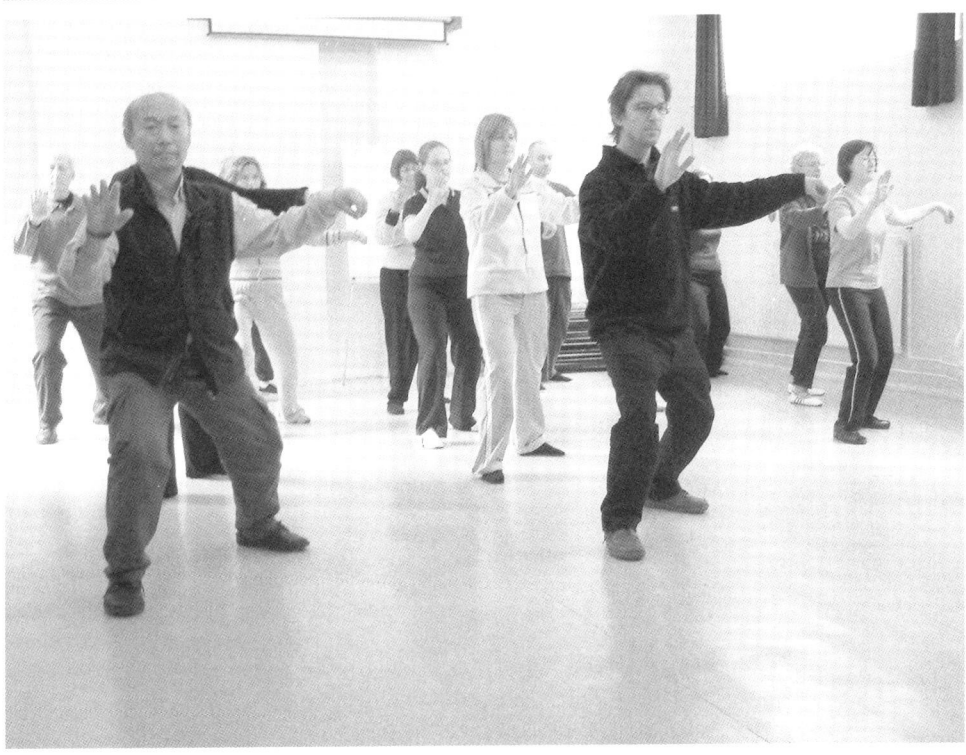

Slow T'ai Chi Form

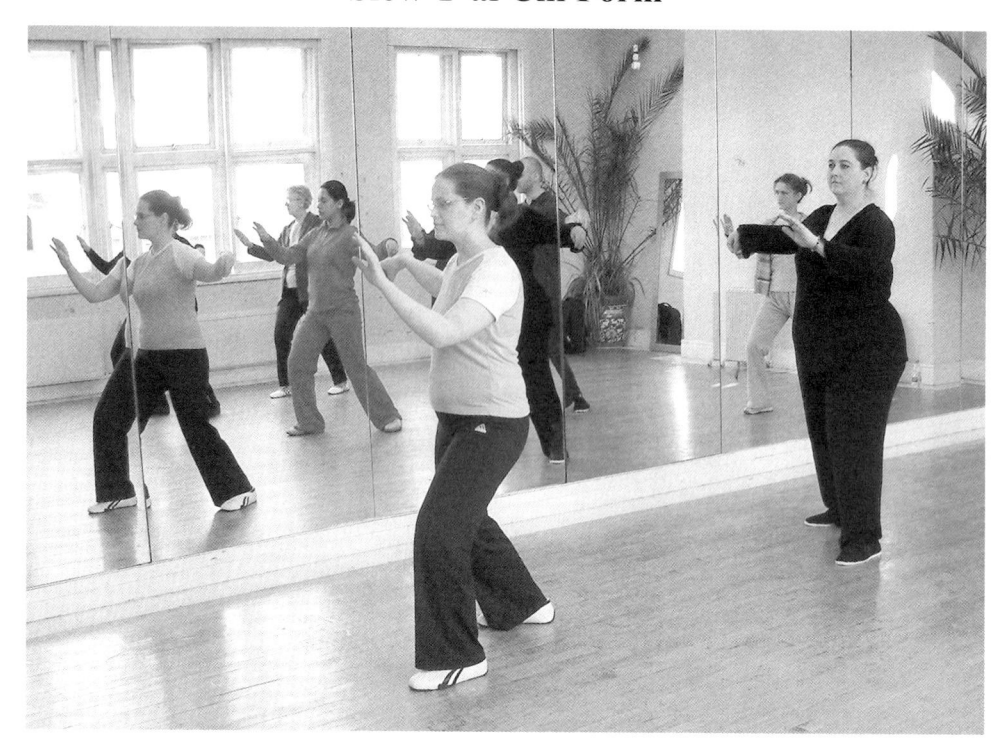

Fast T'ai Chi Form

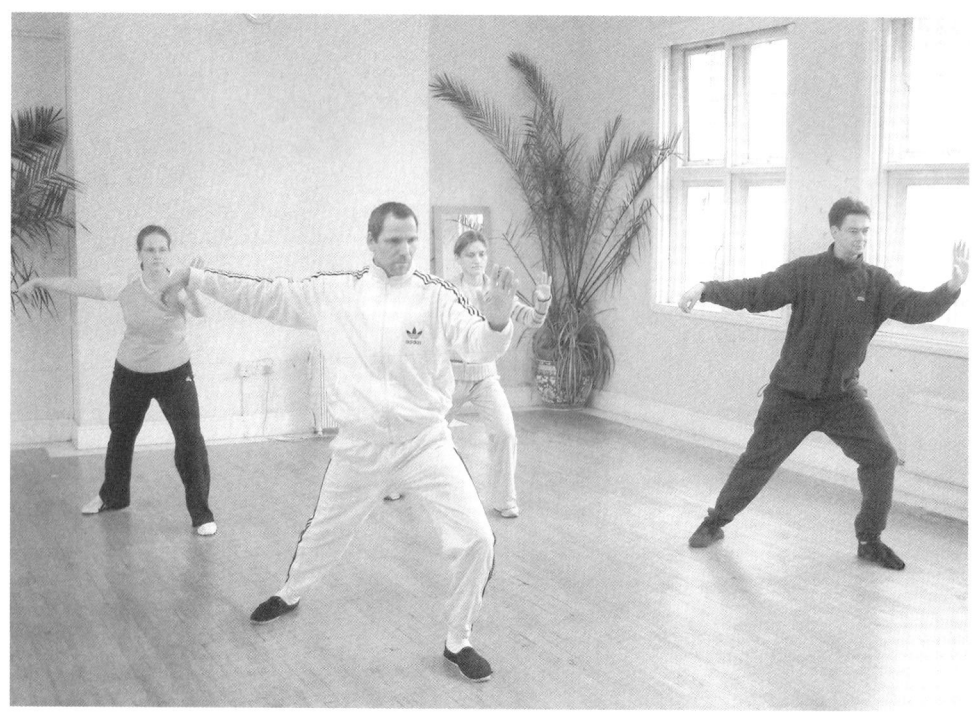

Applied Push Hands

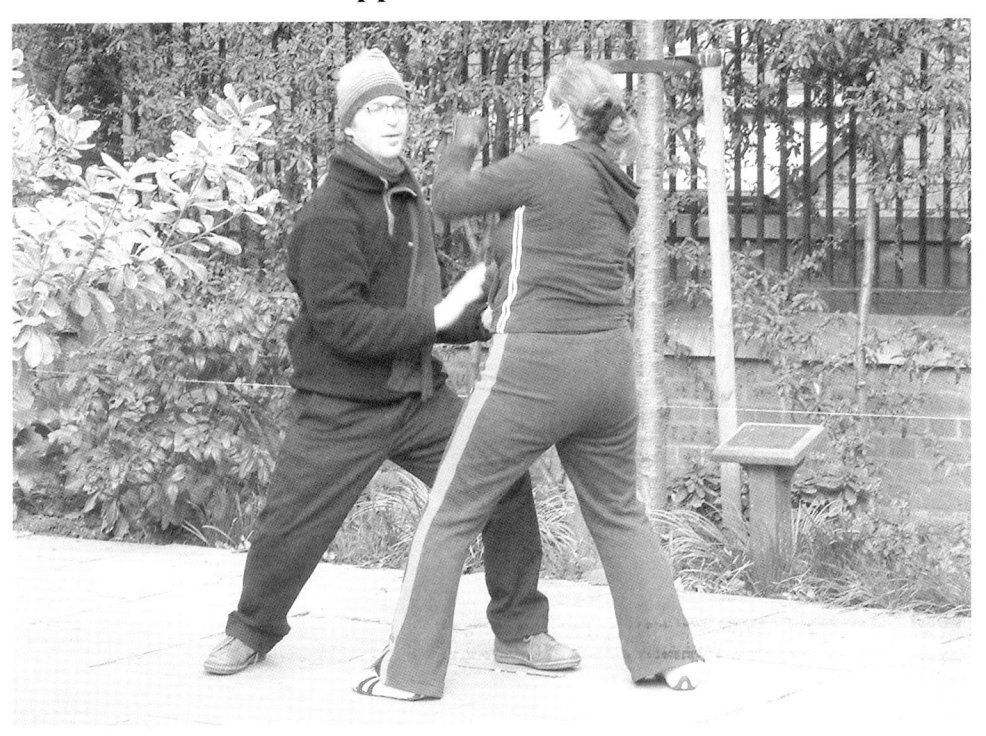

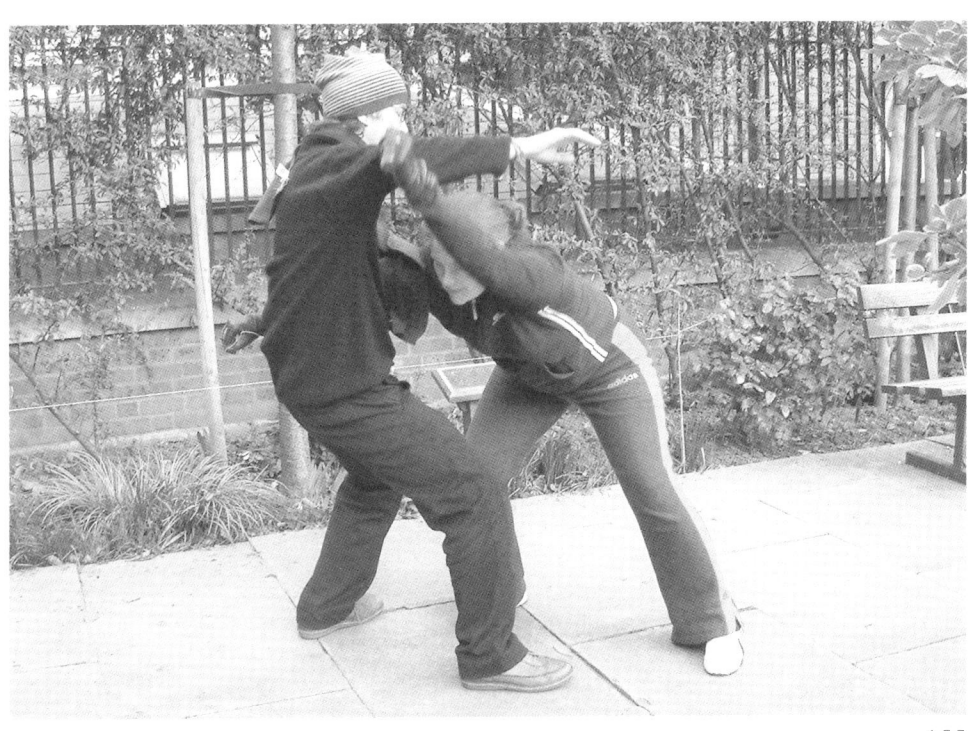

Sword Form

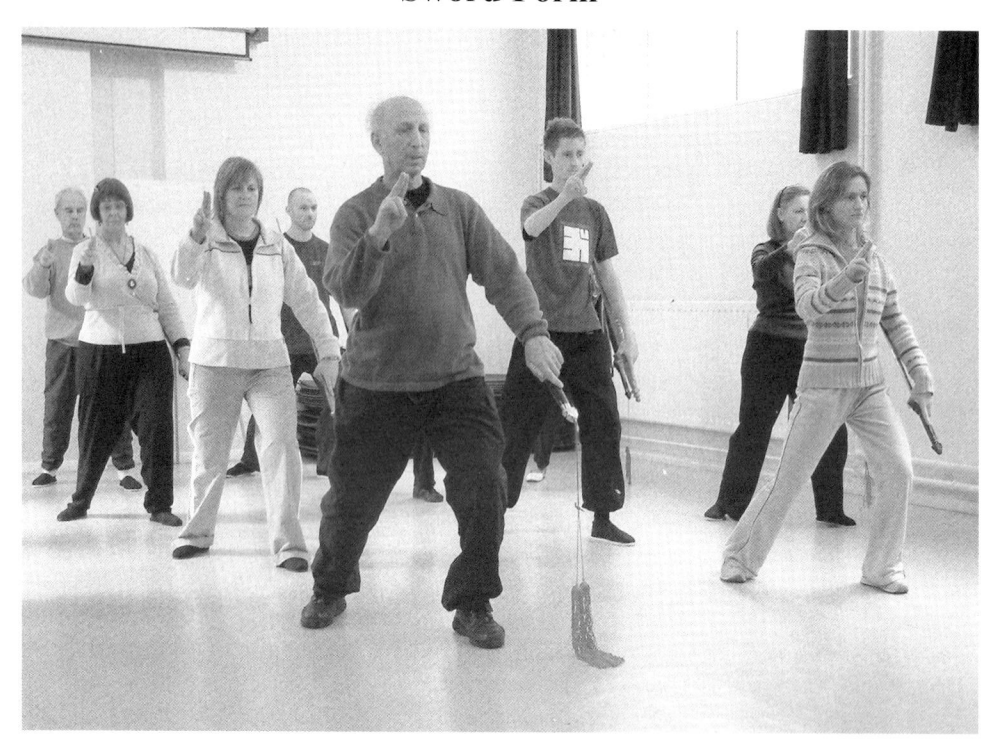

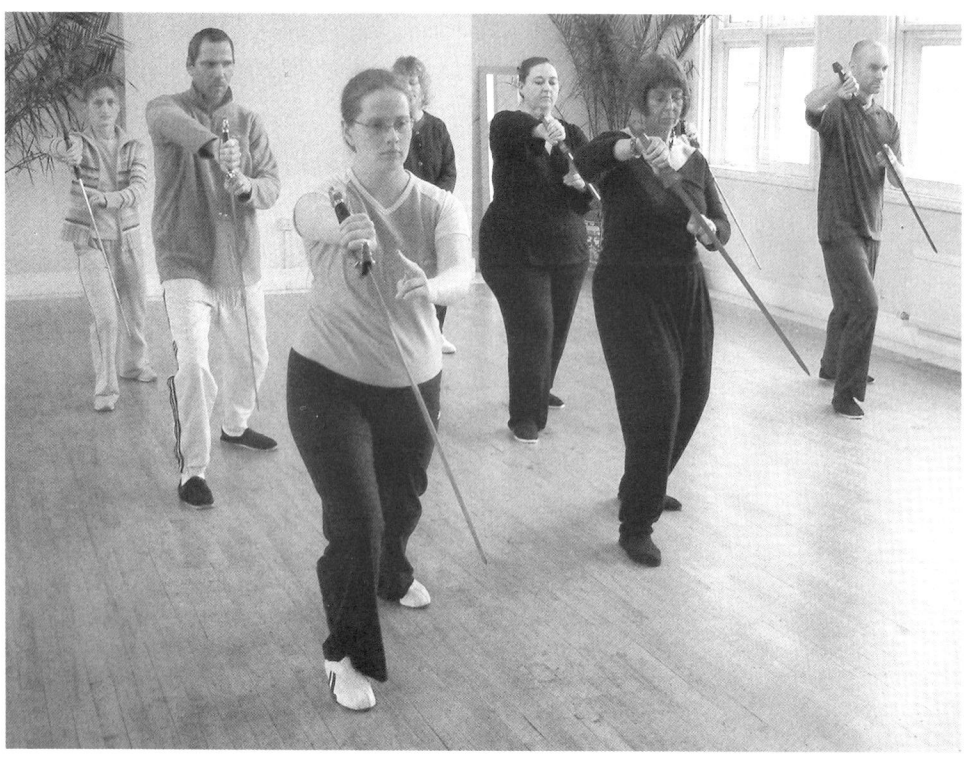

Sword Sparring

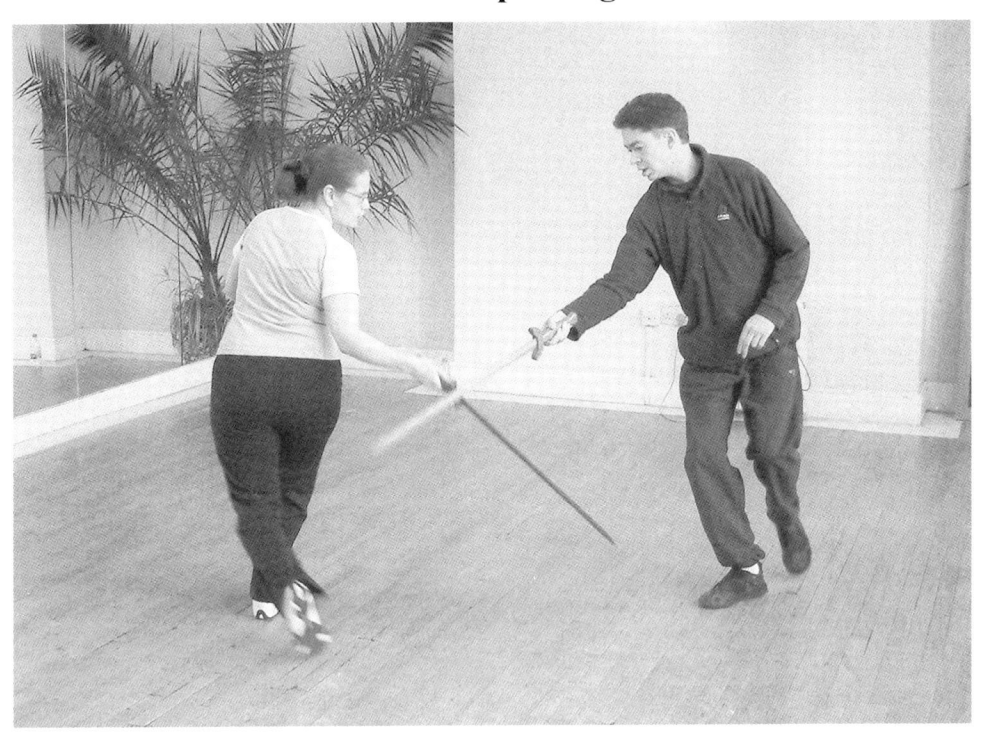

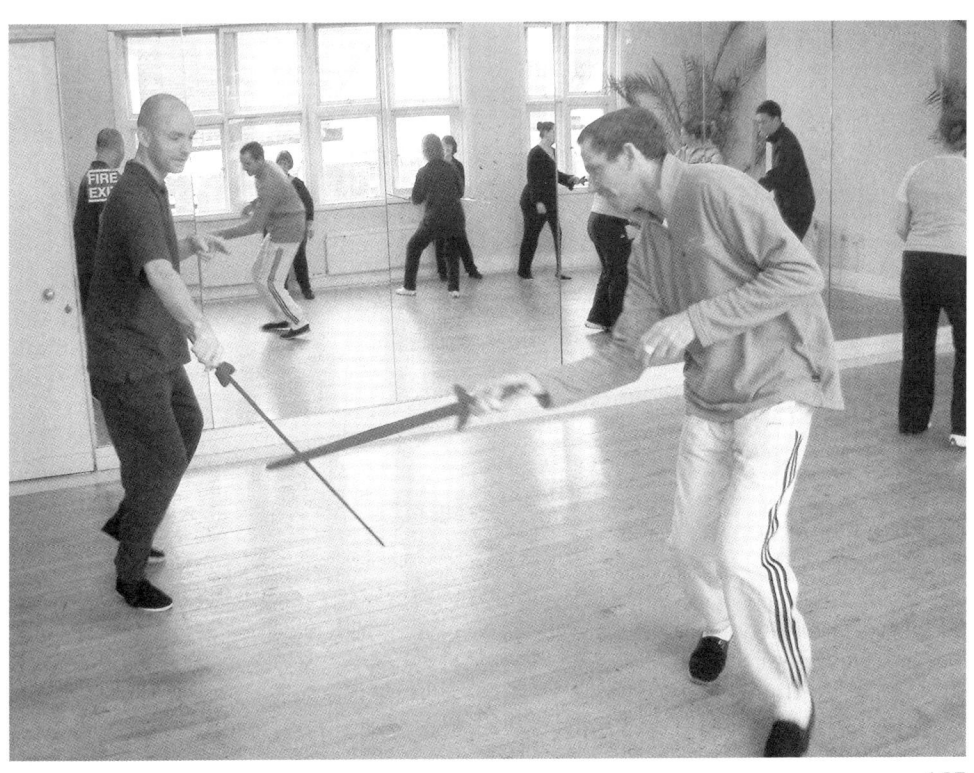

Da Lu

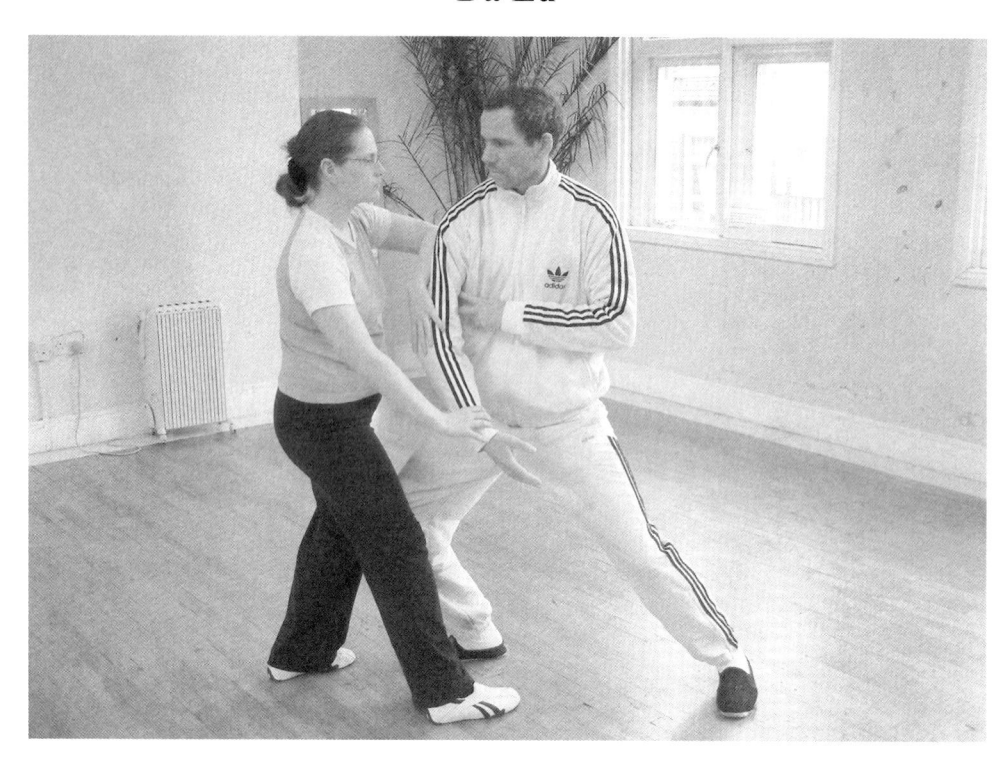

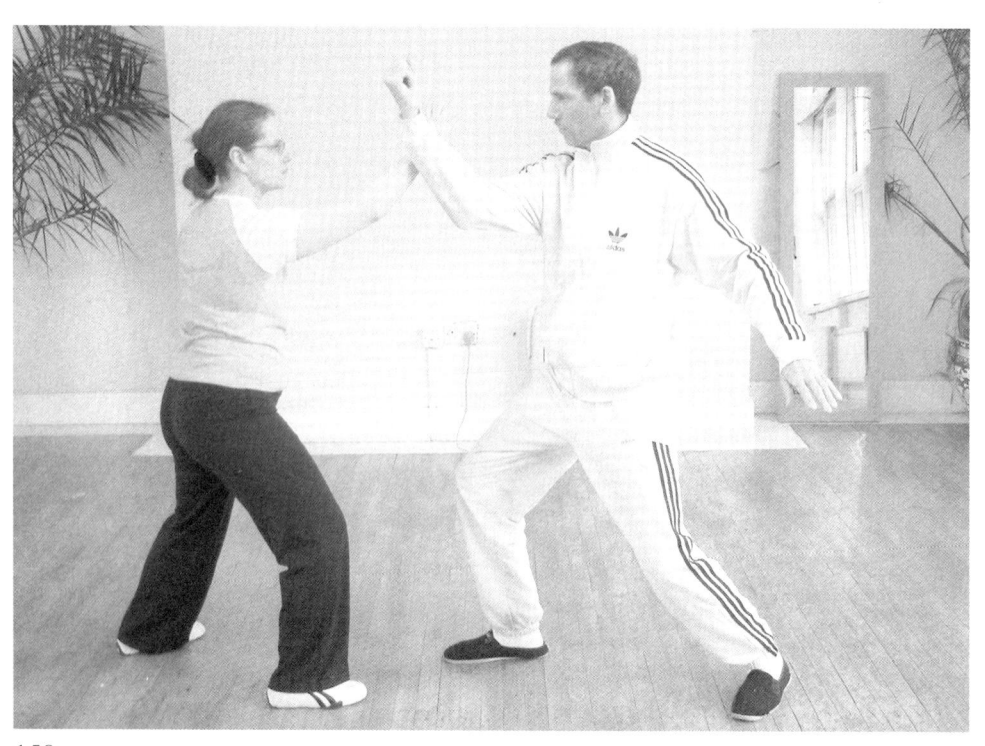

Walking Stick Form

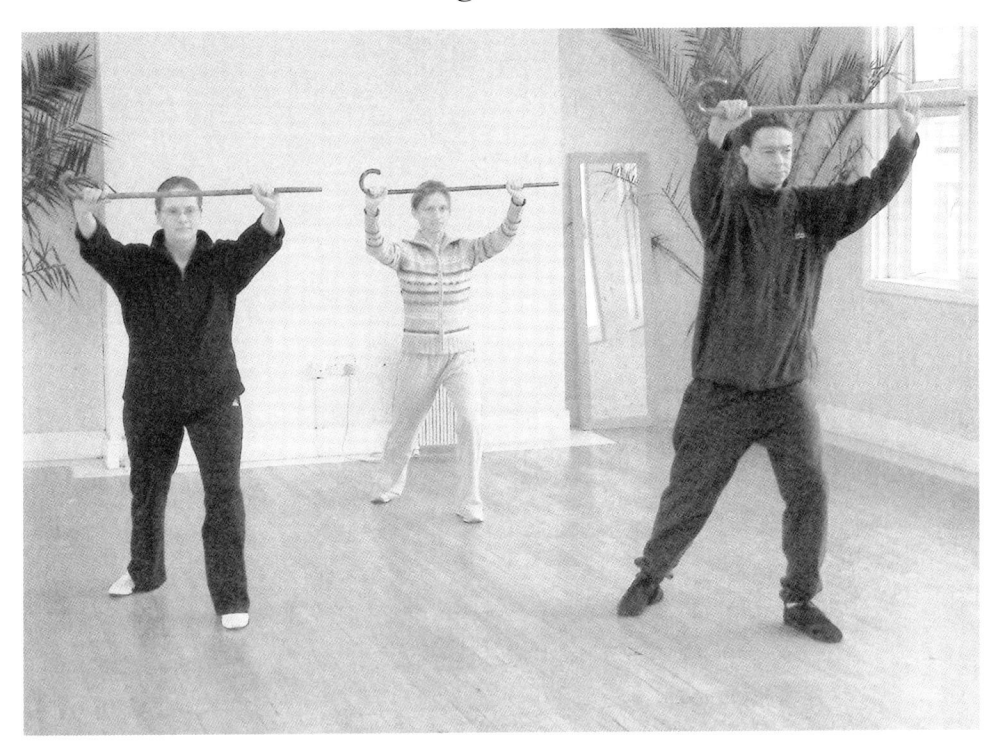

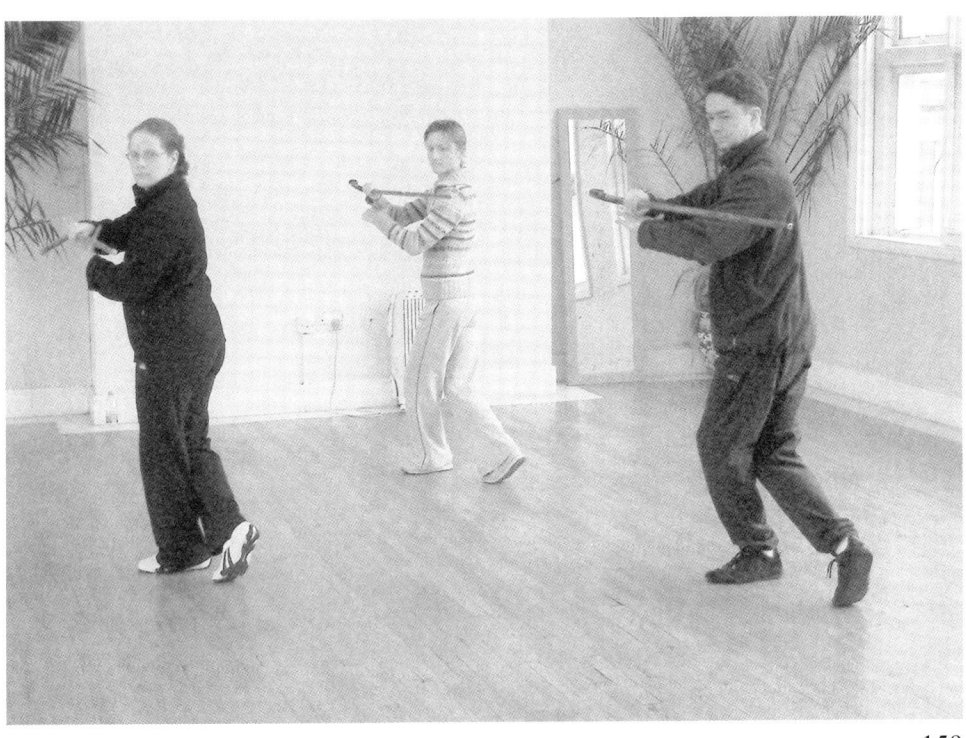

Sabre Form

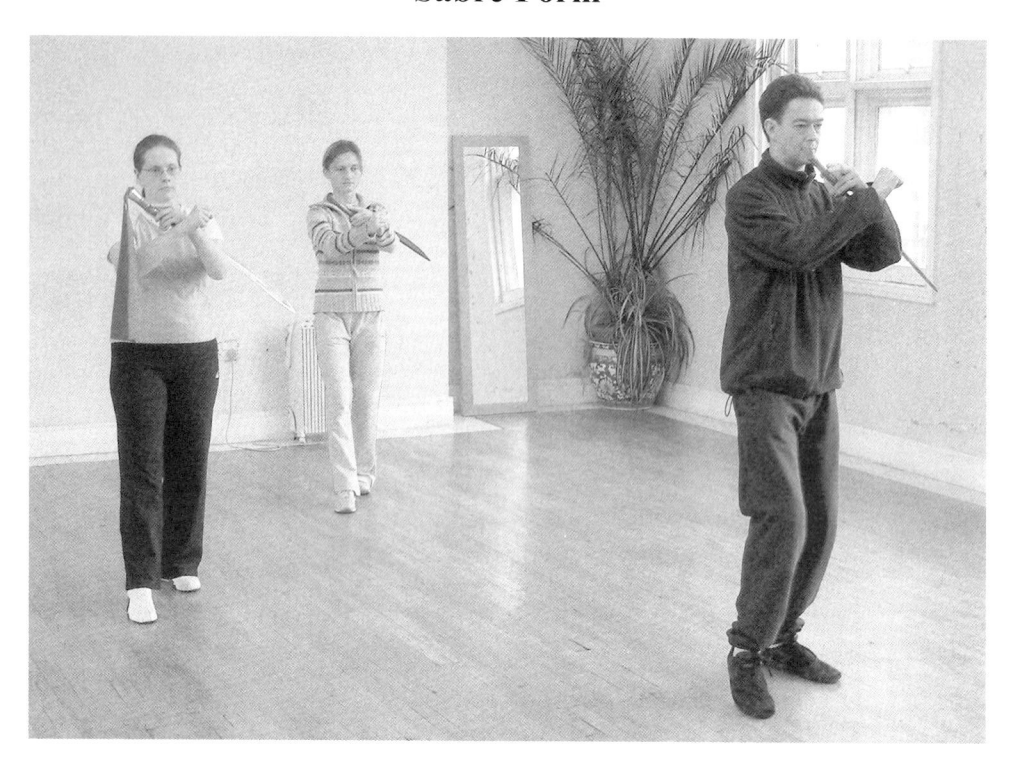

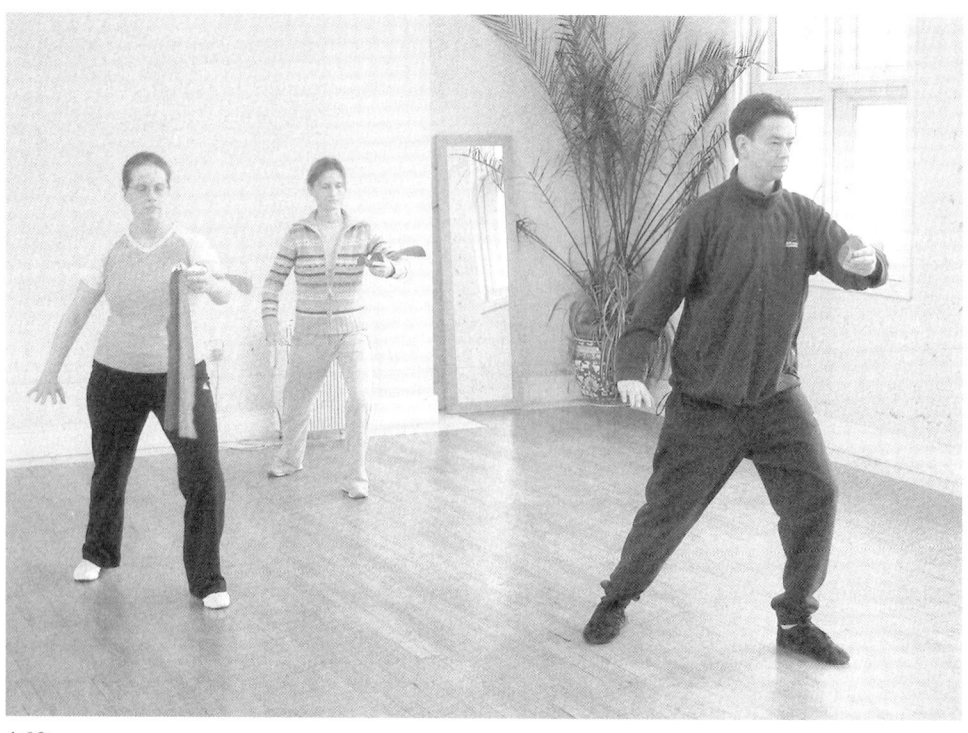

Staff Form

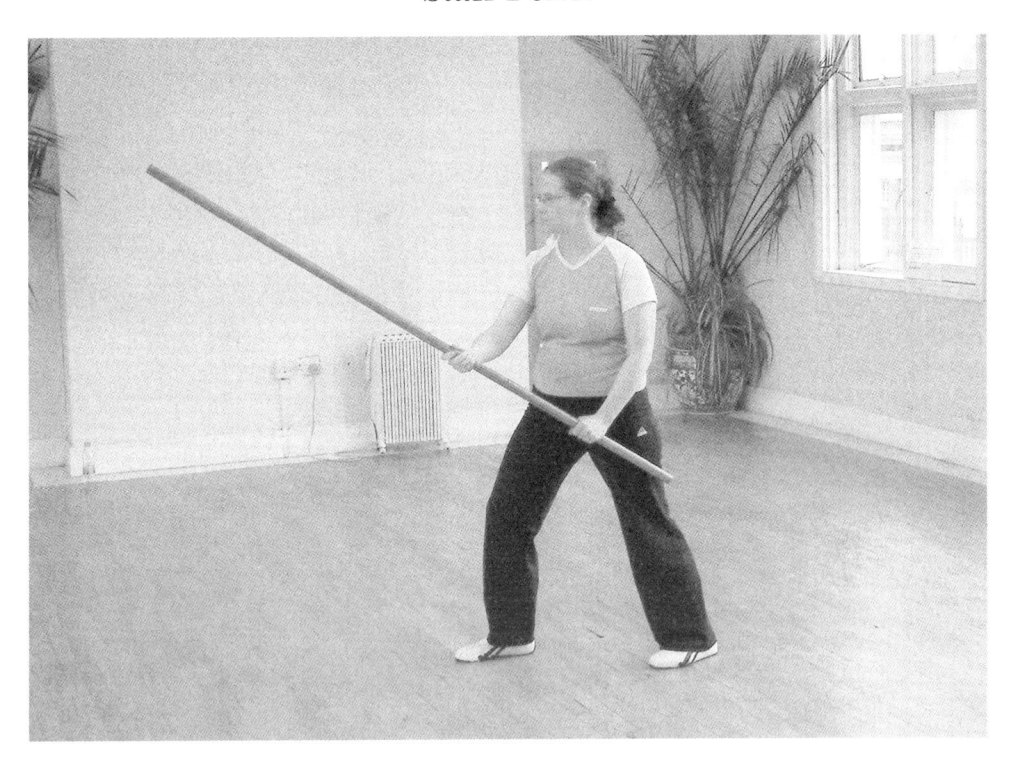

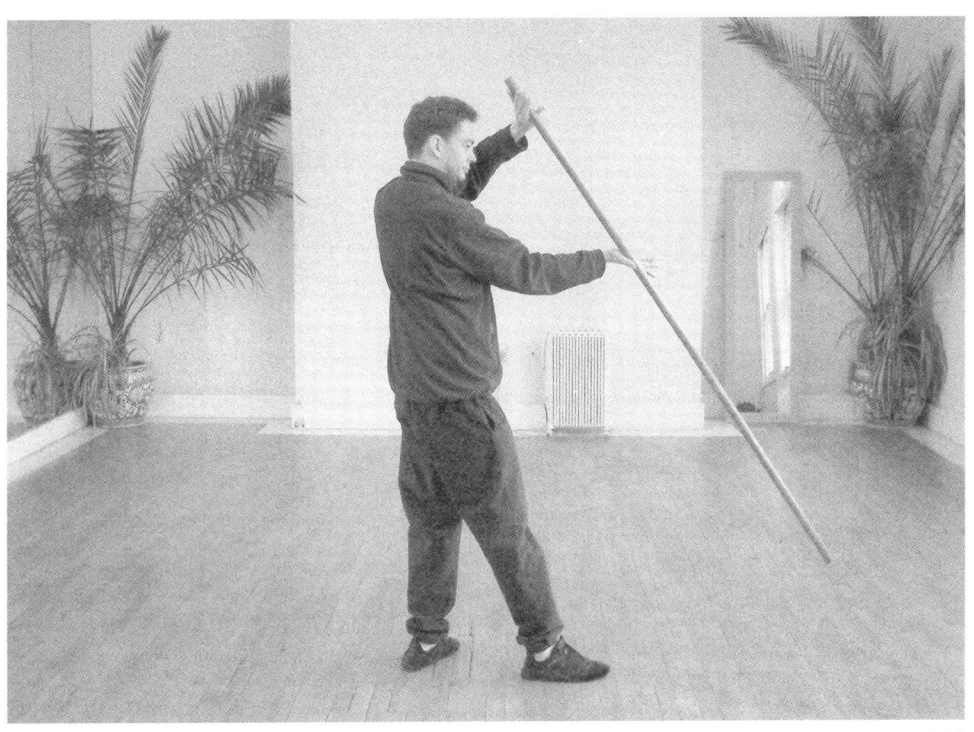

Bag Work

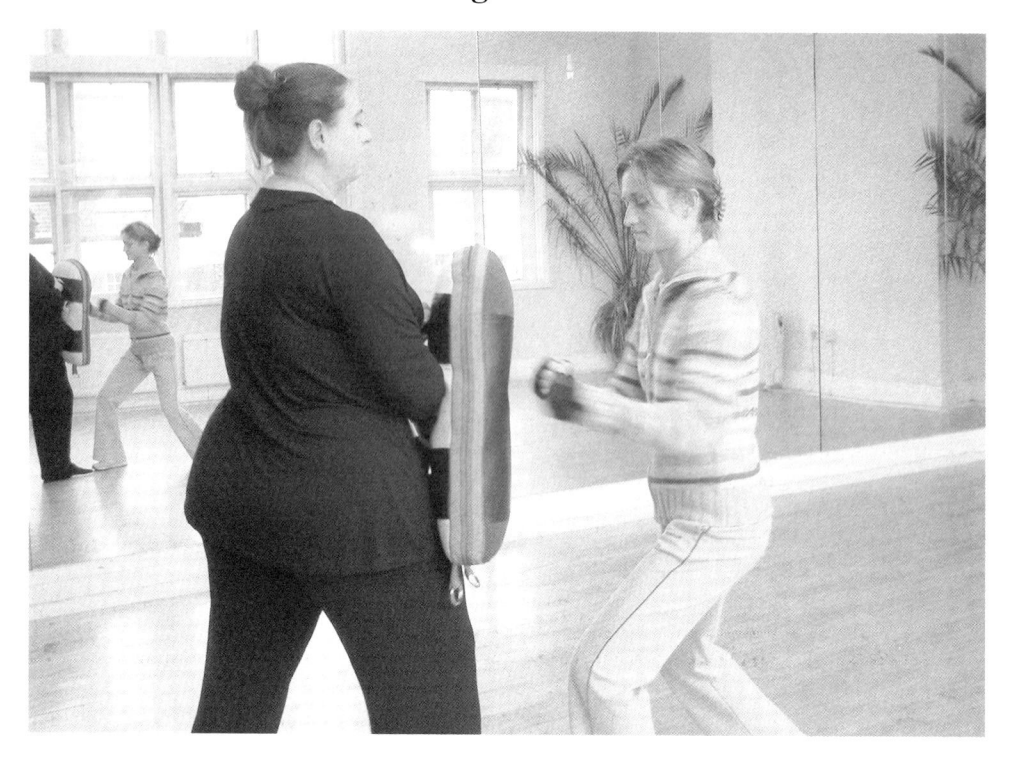

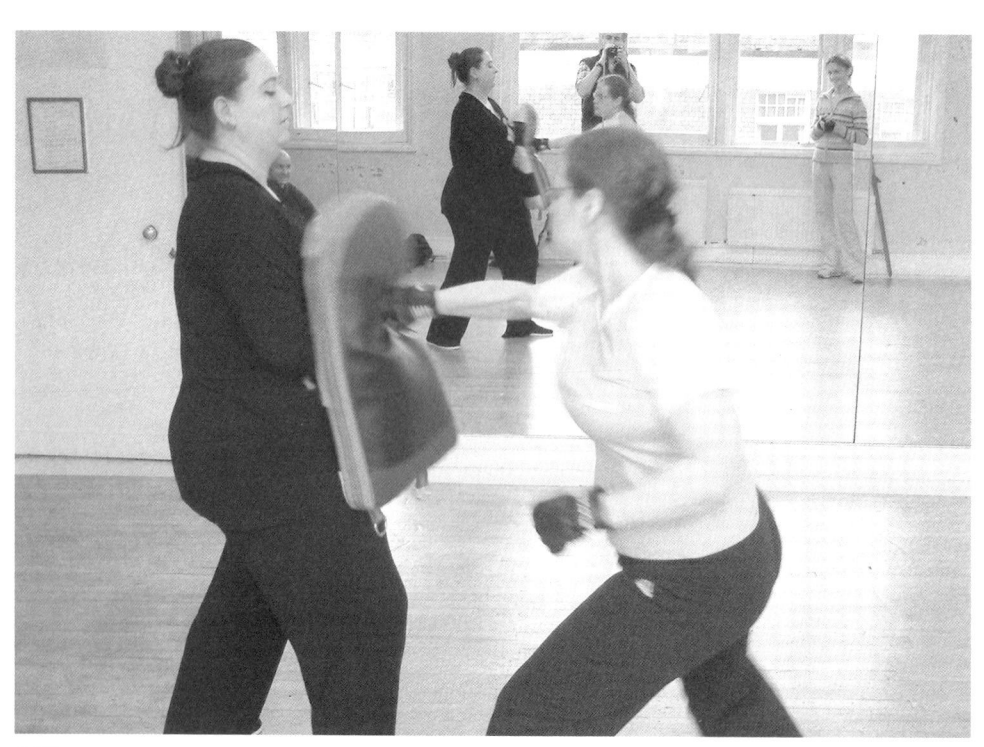

Technique Applications

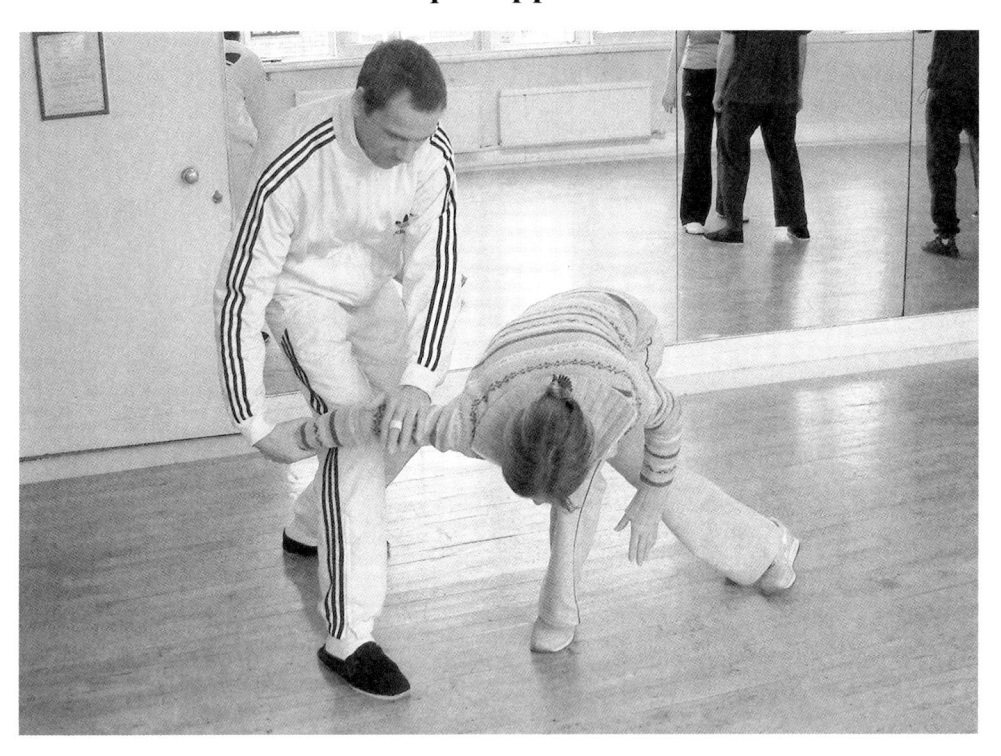

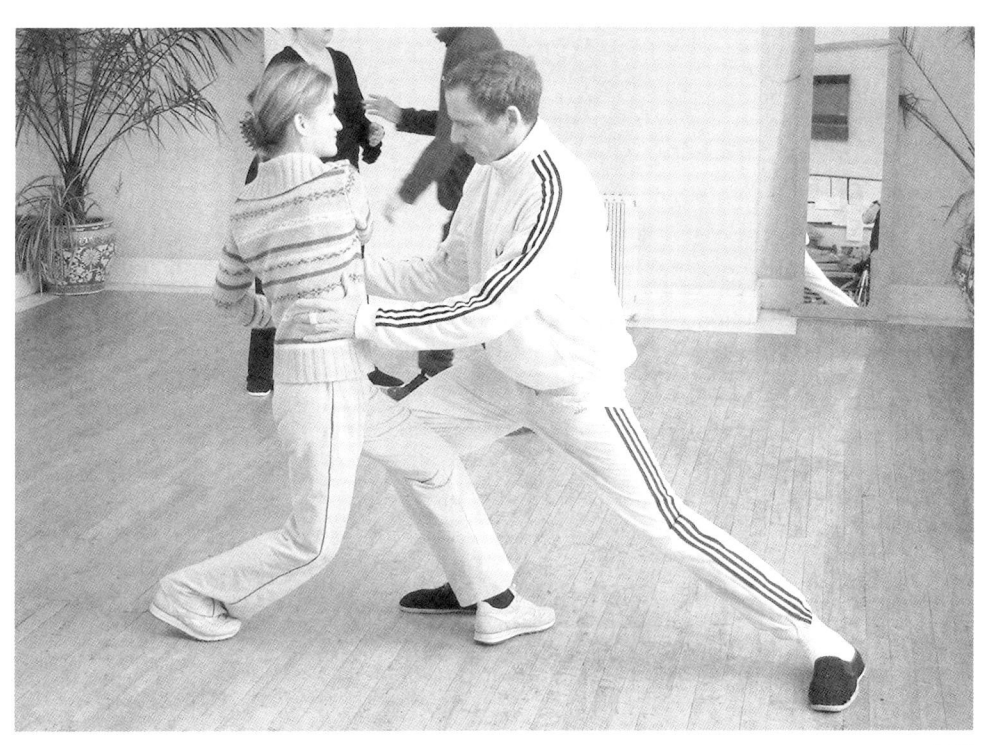

In Conclusion

Energy, ability and capacity are built over time. The state of our minds and bodies will affect our actions. When sufficient action has been taken, the destination will have been reached. There is a saying, 'the path is long but the ox is persistent'. If you stop at any point on your journey from A to B, then you will not get to B. Professor Cheng said that if a technique does not work it means that you have not yet figured out how it works. Insufficient time has been spent practising for the correct outcome to be achieved.

You advance only by taking action. Practice is needed in order to improve at T'ai chi and Chi Kung. Your natural ability and aptitude will be developed with work. You may or may not achieve your full potential but with consistent practice you will have more insight into your potential capacity.

You will advance in your ability by being patient and persistent. Enjoying what you do will make the process more pleasurable. The ancient Taoists aimed to live in harmony with the principles of nature. Their goal was to balance the opposites in their life, what they called the yin and yang. If we can find the appropriate proportion for ourselves then this will affect the quality of our life.

Begin to develop and experience calmness of mind and body. Allow your life to be as stress free as possible. Identify stress factors that interfere with your wellbeing and reduce them and if possible eliminate them. The techniques and forms in this book are practical means for developing mental and physical wellbeing. Once you have the desire for participation in a learning process, it is then a case of sustaining your enthusiasm for learning.

Give yourself gradual, realistic and attainable goals. With repetition you gain improvement and fluency. If you have clear objectives then specific directions are created. Demands create challenges without which growth is not possible. When one becomes clear about what one wants to achieve, then one can better motivate oneself towards success.

It is important to create an environment that is conducive to your own learning. Do not limit your aspirations and work hard. Now is the beginning of your future. What you do now and its quality affects what happens in the future and its quality. The now is so important, nourish it.

If you practise these arts as much as possible you achieve deeper insights into their techniques. You will gain experience and intuitive insight, which will enrich your life as well as others who you share this information with.

Good luck with your practice and training.

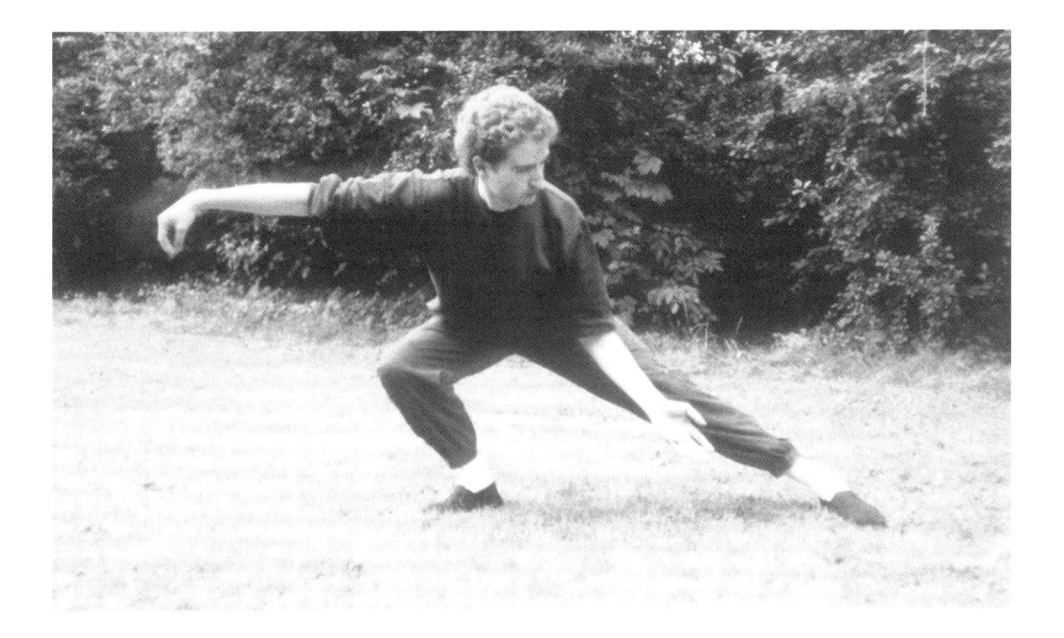

Suggestions for Further Reading

Cheng Man-Ch'ing and Robert W. Smith, 1967, T'ai Chi, The 'Supreme Ultimate' Exercise for Health, Sport and Self-Defense, C E Tuttle Co., Vermont, USA

Cheng Man-Ch'ing, 1981, T'ai Chi Ch'uan, A Simplified Method of Calisthenics for Health & Self Defense, North Atlantic Books, Berkeley, Ca., USA

Cheng Man-Ch'ing, 1982, Master Cheng's Thirteen Chapters on T'ai Chi Ch'uan, Translated by Douglas Wile, Sweet Ch'i Press, N.Y., USA

Cheng Man-Ch'ing, 1985, Cheng Man-Ch'ing's Advanced T'ai Chi Form Instructions, With Selected Writings on Meditation, the I Ching, Medicine and the Arts, Compiled and translated by Douglas Wile, Sweet Ch'i Press, N.Y., USA

Cheng Man-Ch'ing, 1985, Cheng Tzu's Thirteen Treatises on T'ai Chi Ch'uan, Translated by Benjamin Pang Jeng Lo and Martin Inn, North Atlantic Books, Berkeley, Ca., USA

Bibliography

Brookfield, S.D. (1986) Understanding and Facilitating Adult Learning,
Open University, Milton Keynes

Curzon, L.B. (1996) Teaching in Further Education,
Cassell, London

Handley, P. (1973) Personality, Learning and Teaching,
Northumberland Press Ltd., Gateshead

Holms, B. and McLean, M. (1992) The Curriculum - A Comparative Perspective,
Unwin-Hyman, London

Morea, P. (1990) Personality, an Introduction to the Theories of Psychology, Harmondsworth, Penguin Books Ltd.,

Sotto, E. (1997) When Teaching Becomes Learning,
Cassell, London

Dr Yang, J.M. (1989) The Root of Chinese Chi Kung,
YMAA Publications Centre, Jamaica Plain, MA

Zukav, G. (1984) The Dancing Wu Li Masters: An Overview of the New Physics, Flamingo, London

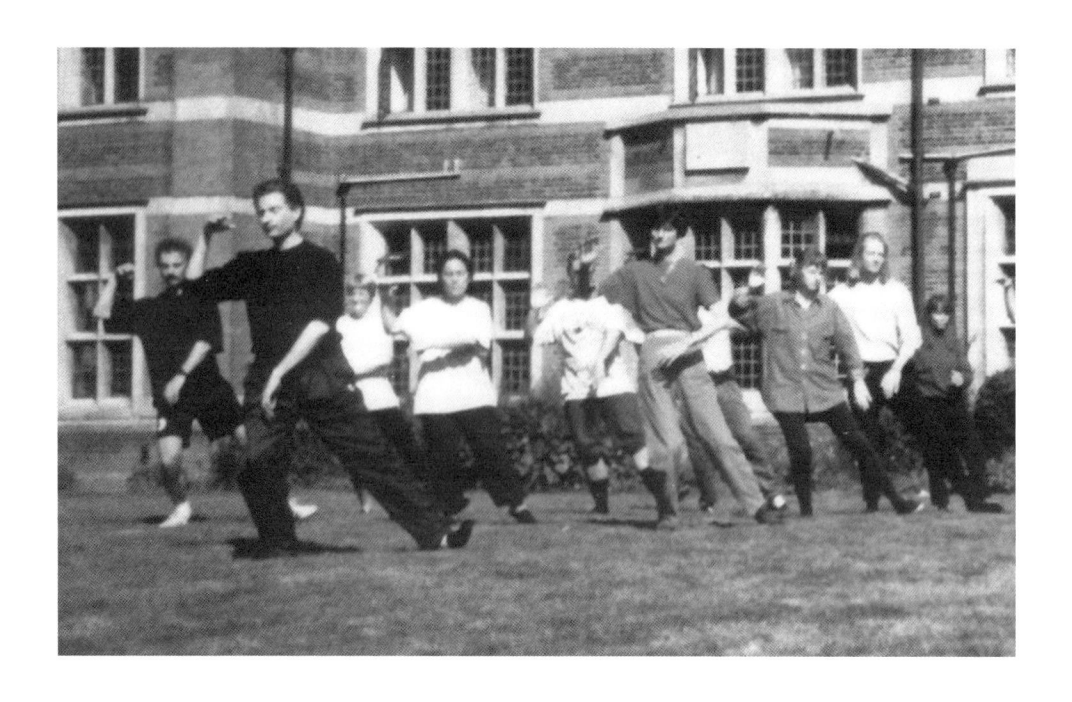

For Further Information Concerning

Classes, Tuition and Retreats
visit our website

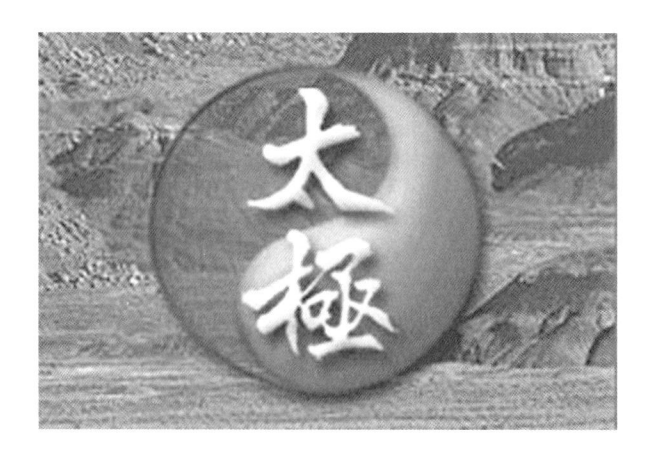

www.vgtaichi.com